In Memoriam

"When from the circling faces, veils pass
And laughing fellowship grows warm"
Arthur Davison Ficke

**Peter Canty, Paule Cotter, Dermot Crean, Des Kelleher,
Barney Nagle, John O'Connell, Denis O'Connor, Mary O'Connor,
Jim O'Driscoll, Tim O'Herlihy**

Liberating the Butterfly

The butterfly represents celebration of life through venturesome living.
It corresponds to Antonovsky's use of heterostasis as the underlying spirit of
salutogenesis.

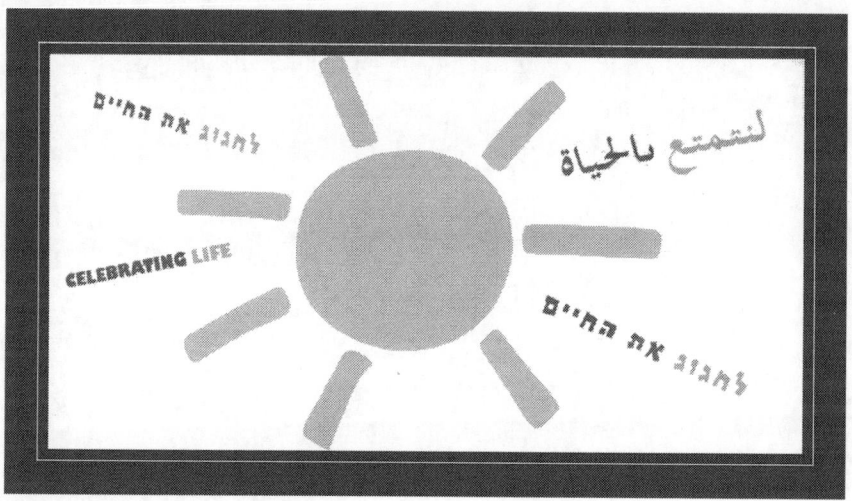

Photo taken at entrance to Jordan River Valley, the Serious Fun camp in Israel.

Healing Rites of Passage

This book examines how 'Therapeutic Recreation' transforms the social health of children enduring or recovering from life-threatening illnesses such as cancer and leukaemia. With studies drawn from 'Serious Fun' projects in the USA, the UK, France, Ireland and Israel, the author explores how camp experiences in convivial circumstances help to bring about healing. Employing central concepts from sociology and anthropology, such as 'liminality', 'mimesis' and 'salutogenesis', *Healing Rites of Passage* explains why a brief secluded holiday can reform the campers' shared situation of life-threatening illnesses towards health and flourishing. The whole process can be understood in terms of a 'rite of passage', as structured camp experiences enable children to shed previous 'sick roles' and pass through a series of challenges in order to achieve social re-integration with a renewed zest for living. An empirically grounded study that reveals the analytical value of master concepts in the social sciences, this book will appeal to scholars in the fields of sociology, anthropology, paediatrics, social theory and the sociology of health, illness and medicine.

Peter James Kearney is Emeritus Professor of Paediatrics and Occasional Lecturer in Sociology at University College Cork, Ireland.

The Social Pathologies of Contemporary Civilization

Edited by Anders Petersen, Kieran Keohane and Bert van den Bergh

Breaking decisively with the often ideological and moralistic approach of treating problems of health and well-being as discrete and individual problems to be addressed in isolation both from one another and their broader social contexts, this series pursues the investigation of the ways in which contemporary malaises, diseases, illnesses and psychosomatic syndromes are related to cultural pathologies of the social body and disorders of the collective ésprit de corps of contemporary society.

It avoids reductive psychological and biomedical understandings of pathologies – including depression, stress-related illnesses, eating disorders, suicide and deliberate self-harm – to focus instead on the socio-cultural contexts in which they occur, examining the radical changes to social structures and institutions, and the deep crises in our civilization as a whole to which such conditions are connected.

The Social Pathologies of Contemporary Civilization thus welcomes manuscripts from a broad range of disciplinary perspectives across the humanities and social sciences – sociology, philosophy, psychology, anthropology, politics, economics and cultural studies, as well as from the fields of medicine social care, therapeutic practice and the healing arts – that explore the fruitfulness locating health and well-being not simply in the individual body or soul, but within a trans-disciplinary imagination that takes into account the integral human person's situatedness within collective social bodies, particular communities, entire societies, or even whole civilizations.

Titles in the series

Late Modern Subjectivity and its Discontents
Anxiety, Depression and Alzheimer's Disease
Kieran Keohane, Anders Petersen and Bert van den Bergh

States of Intoxication
The Place of Alcohol in Civilisation
John O'Brien

Healing Rites of Passage
Salutogenesis in Serious Fun Camps
Peter James Kearney

For more information about this series, please visit: https://www.routledge.com/ The-Social-Pathologies-of-Contemporary-Civilization/book-series/ASHSER1434

Healing Rites of Passage

Salutogenesis in Serious Fun Camps

Peter James Kearney

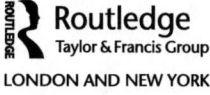

Routledge
Taylor & Francis Group

LONDON AND NEW YORK

First published 2019
by Routledge
2 Park Square, Milton Park, Abingdon, Oxon OX14 4RN

and by Routledge
52 Vanderbilt Avenue, New York, NY 10017

First issued in paperback 2020

Routledge is an imprint of the Taylor & Francis Group, an informa business

British Library Cataloguing-in-Publication Data
A catalogue record for this book is available from the British Library

Library of Congress Cataloging-in-Publication Data
A catalog record has been requested for this book

ISBN 13: 978-0-36-758507-5 (pbk)
ISBN 13: 978-0-415-79124-3 (hbk)

Typeset in Bembo
by codeMantra

Contents

Acknowledgements

This book would not have happened but for local circumstances in Cork necessitating my return to Paediatric Oncology in the Children's Leukaemia Unit of the Mercy University Hospital, where I first witnessed the magic of the Barretstown experience. The late Séamus O'Donoghue, Michael Madden and the Paediatric Oncology Nurses had set up a deeply caring unit, which made practice there very satisfying. I am indebted to Kieran Keohane who was the accoucheur that supervised delivery of this book after a long gestation. He was also my guide to Sociology and a great interpreter of inchoate ideas. Kieran pointed out to me early on while still a practising Paediatrician that my interest in Barretstown was about Social Transformations. The book would not have been written without the constant care and support of Siún, who gave unstinting encouragement and, as the book took shape, was an incisive reader reflecting her interests in social work, law and mediation. Our daughters Fiona, Patricia, Oonagh and Siún Ann, and my brother Kevin in the USA all cast critical eyes over the text. Terry Kelleher knew better than most that 'perfection is the enemy of success' – an underlying theme of the book. Terry was a film producer and journalist of distinction. He died of multiple sclerosis after a long struggle, just before I could send him a PDF for comment. He is a missing reader buried at sea near Tyrella, Coosheen (another land in a small cove, anglicised from the Irish *Tír Eile, Cuasín*). My medical reader was my old friend and classmate John Good. John O'Brien from Waterford Institute of Technology gave sound advice from a sociological perspective. I am deeply grateful to them all. When I write I think of medieval poets who signed themselves as Anon for they were aware that their writings were only an expression of crucial social experiences.

My introduction to Serious Fun camps was in Barretstown, Co. Kildare, Ireland, by Terry Dignan and I am indebted to him and his deep knowledge of the needs of children in camp. Interviews with different staff in Barretstown, the Painted Turtle and the Hole in the Wall Gang Camps over several years were crucial in developing my understanding of how the camp operates and its effect on seriously ill children. It was a pleasure to work with many colleagues in the Med Shed over the years, which always ran smoothly under the leadership of Eimear Kinsella. My Paediatric colleagues Peter Barbor and

Alfonso Rodríguez were like me intrigued and puzzled by Barretstown and I thank them for their perspectives. Peter Hanlon and Suzie Guerin contributed helpful observations from their development of bereavement camps in Barretstown. The most enlightening insights came from group interviews with camp alumni from Barretstown and the Painted Turtle. I am most grateful to the Caras in Barretstown and the Counselors in the Painted Turtle who likewise communicated the effect of Serious Fun camps not only on the children but also on themselves.

I thank Nancy Scheper Hughes in Berkeley, who helped me negotiate the intricacies of the University of California Committee for the Protection of Human Subjects; Jimmy Canton, Matt Cooke and Karen Carlson of the Hole in the Wall Gang Camp, Connecticut; Blake Maher, Ben Meisel, Jessica Santos and Jeremy Zinger of the Painted Turtle, California.

I am very grateful to the anonymous reviewers who correctly identified a weak conclusion, which I have now expanded. Neil Jordan and Alice Salt of Routledge, and Emeline Jarvie of Codemantra were excellent communicators and gave very constructive advice.

Series editor's foreword

On the face of it, this book, the subject matter of which is childhood, play and *joie de vivre*, does not appear to be about the social pathologies of contemporary civilisation or even about 'social' pathology at all, for leukaemia and other life-threatening illnesses afflicting the children whom we meet in this book are not social pathologies but biomedical pathologies. However, what is remarkable is that while their pathologies are not social in origin, the key to these children's full and successful recovery is very much grounded in anthropological, social, cultural and civilisational factors. Our hope for *Social Pathologies of Contemporary Civilization* as a research project and as a book series is to develop a 'sociotherapy' to correspond with our diagnostics of social pathologies, and this book leads us in just such a hopeful direction.

This beautiful study in applied salutogenesis reflects the author's background as a medical doctor. Peter Kearney was Professor of Paediatric Medicine with a specialism in oncology when, late in his career, he ran up against the limits of the biomedical paradigm in explaining the phenomenon he analyses here: sick children who attended 'Serious Fun' camps have, later in life, a strikingly better recovery experience than children who were equally sick, and who survived, but who did not attend these camps. The children who go to Serious Fun camps re-enter the stream of life and go on to flourish, or at least to lead normal lives; whereas children who do not may not ever fully recover, and many live damaged lives, marked by their childhood illness: they are risk-averse, overcautious and do not flourish. The effect is empirically real and clinically observable, but there is no biomedical explanation for it.

The core of this lucid book, which discloses its profound insights with ease and grace, is an illustration, application and elaboration of Aron Antonovsky's paradigm-shifting concept of salutogenesis, in that Peter Kearney's analysis and interpretation of the therapeutic effects of the 'Serious Fun' camp experience not only solve an enigmatic conundrum that previously seemed inexplicable or 'miraculous', but in solving that mystery he effects a genuine breakthrough, because his analysis has ramifications for our understanding of sickness, treatment, recovery and well-being far beyond this immediate case. What are the implications of this analysis of salutogenesis in Serious Fun camps for, let us say, depression, and so many other maladies of the soul of modern society that we are formulating in this book series in terms of their being Social Pathologies of Contemporary Civilization? We – at least some of us! – know that the biomedical understanding and pharmaceutical treatment of depression is spurious and ineffective, and that it probably perpetuates more illness than it 'cures'. A typical trajectory is 'diagnosis' of a 'disease' that is then 'managed' by 'medication' over a long term – very often 'lifelong' – without the person ever properly 'recovering' at all, so that they are trapped perpetually in a liminal grey zone: the stigmatised, numbed, half-life of a 'person living with depression'.

Biomedical pharma-psychiatry is very much part of the problem rather than a solution to the social pathologies of contemporary civilization, and so too, but for a different though closely related reason, are the problems associated with various genres of clinical 'talk therapy'. Most obvious is Cognitive Behavioural Therapy, because it is so patently shallow, 'managing' symptoms without addressing their sources; but psychotherapeutic counselling and psychoanalysis too, with frequent stories of 'clients' becoming trapped in lifelong dependent, often exploitative relationships with 'therapists', their analysis 'going nowhere', just like the 'patients' who develop dependencies on addictive anti-depressants and their doctors who prescribe them and the corporate pharmaceuticals giants that are pushing them. The paradigm that Medicine shares with Psychology, and the limitation that they share in common, is that they are both reductively individualistic: just as bio-psychiatry is individually reductive to neurochemistry, the problem with the clinical talk therapies is that they are, to a greater or lesser degree, reductive to the individual's psychology and personality.

Here, with Peter Kearney's book, we have something genuinely new: for the children who participate in Serious Fun camps, the trajectory of disease and the outcome of treatment is known and predictable in the sense that if medical treatment succeeds the child lives, if it fails then the child dies. But what is not known, and what seems enigmatic and 'magical' is the difference in the trajectory of recovery: of those children who survive, some of them go on to live much better than others, and the key difference in determining successful recovery from psychological injuries associated with life-threatening illness (the trauma of effective but aggressive treatment including painful surgeries and chemotherapies; the existential terror of exposure to death; the loneliness of extended hospitalisation; the disruption of childhood; loss of peers; deep, protracted, lingering stigma; and so on) is by a structured intervention that is *sociotherapeutic*.

The sociotherapy that Peter Kearney's analysis of salutogenesis in Serious Fun camps brings to light entails a deliberate and systematically organised structuring of the experience of recovering a sense of coherence and re-entering the stream of life, and that structured experience is derived from anthropologically deep-seated and socially universal forms, namely: the *rite de passage* as a cohort experience of progressive status elevation and social re-integration (Arnold van Gennip and Victor Turner); mimetic desire to emulate models (Rene Girard); and the integration of these corpora of anthropological theory to sociologically formulate the pathogenic condition of Modernity as permanent liminality (Arpad Szakolczai). The principles of the sociotherapy that Peter Kearney synthesises and distills from these conceptual elements can potentially be applied and extended into other illnesses, and into clinical therapies and rehabilitative practices, and not just for children, but throughout the life course. How could our understanding of and our treatment of depression, anxiety, anorexia, or so many other malaises that we argue are social pathologies of contemporary civilization be transformed if viewed in the light of the sociotherapy suggested here?

We will all find ourselves, at some stage of our life course, to have become 'citizens in the state of the unwell', as Susan Sontag calls it, experiencing complexes of physical and mental suffering with devastating social–psychological impacts. The person with severe depression, for instance, typically experiences disruption of social relations; loss of colleagues, friends, family and partner; stigma; loss of social status; loss of face; loss of self-esteem and self-confidence; dejection and existential dread; numbness, as well as generalised anxiety and terror. Being a citizen of the state of the unwell entails a comprehensive fragmentation of the previously taken-for-grantedness of the person's shared symbolic universe, leading to loss of meaningfulness, asymbolia and absurdity, the deep wellsprings of pathogenesis in contemporary civilisation.

Recovery from such states of unwellness may be better effected not by medication, or not even by individual talk therapy, but rather by a salutogenic sociotherapy that systematically sets about repairing the very tissue of social life, that is to say repairing the symbolic order and the imaginative texture of the person's life-world. The 'active ingredients', so to speak, for such a sociotherapy may be found already present and close to hand in civilisationally deep-seated collective knowledge, anthropologically encoded in the meaning-making structure of ritual, elementary forms of healthful and meaningful life that may be derived and distilled by analysis, and, with imagination and care, can be re-formulated into institutions and practices to enable a deliberate re-symbolisation, ritually 'suturing' the person back into the symbolic order, first as a member of a cohort sharing a common pathologic situation, re-configured as a salutogenic experience of progressive status elevation, towards their re-integration into a meaningful whole.

The [further] problem is, unfortunately, that the 'meaningful whole' that is society is seriously damaged (and damaging; indeed the source of the individual's damage in the first place!) due to 'de-symbolisation', as analysed by the cultural socioanalyst Dany-Robert Dufour, 'social acceleration', as formulated by the sociologist Hartmut Rosa, and other generalised historical effects of the postmodern condition and the neoliberal revolution. But even these macro-level sources of pathogenesis could be addressed by an anthropologically grounded sociotherapy that Peter Kearney's analysis of the 'Serious Fun' camp experience gives us a first glimpse of. Just as the *rite de passage* typically entails initiation into 'sacred mysteries' guided by wise and caring masters of ceremonies, the mysteries revealed through a sociotherapy for addressing the social pathologies of contemporary civilization might be thought of in terms of an initiation into the Girardian and the Derridean/Lacanian mystery of the Lack; the Real; those 'things hidden since the foundation of the world', that is, the obscure, unstable grounds of the entire edifice of civilisation that are the source of humankind's insatiable desire for order and our perpetual search for meaning in the face of the fragility and precarity of life, and the constitutionally flawed nature of the symbolic order, in general, and the fatal flaws of the symbolic orders of the present in particular. Such a revealing, not of an 'internal' flaw in the subject's cognition or in their personal biography, but of an 'external' flaw in prevailing social structures, may itself be not just therapeutic in relieving the person of the burden of responsibility for their suffering, but even emancipatory, in the sense suggested by the author of *Civilization and its Discontents* that 'to be sane in a sick society is to be sick relative to the society!'

Peter Kearney brings Antonovsky's concept of salutogenesis into harmony, so to speak, with Hartmut Rosa's concept of 'resonance'. Late Modernity ignores and denies human limits at the cost of anthropological grounds of sustainable life on one hand and transcendental ideals on the other. Relations of resonance between ideals and grounds refer to phenomena that are 'vague', that is relations that are intangible, immeasurable, but that are absolutely concrete, basic: such things are the moral foundations of society. Lacking resonant relations between grounds and limits, loss of moral centre and anchorage, our lives and minds become unstrung. We oscillate wildly, distuned, a violent cacophony. The isolist subjectivity towards which contemporary neoliberal civilisation is moving us has destructive effects in all sorts of ways. If one puts the key concept of salutogenesis – 'sense of coherence' (esp. 'meaningfulness') – in the light of this isolism, then it becomes a counter-concept, counter-movement, counter-ideology, counter-strategy or whatever one might name it. In the register of musical metaphor suggested by Rosa's concept of resonance, salutogenesis is a 'counter-point' to the discordance and dissonance associated with neoliberal isolism. As a case study of 'disconnecting in order to reconnect' the rite de passage as a bridge to a new or renewed connection, coherence, meaningfulness shows us a direction back to life, to life's rhythmicity, to the rhythmic whole of life, to a renewed and elementary salutogenic 'sense of coherence'.

Pathogenesis and salutogenesis are two sides of the same coin. Jacques Schotte, the Belgian psychiatrist/psychoanalyst, calls his approach 'pathoanalysis': the analysis of pathology leads to an understanding of the basis of human existence. If 'isolism' lies at the heart of contemporary social pathologies, then 'sense of coherence' is a concept that opens up the path towards our main remedy: pathoanalysis, salutogenesis, sociotherapy: a divine trinity! This book, which, of course, in the first instance, is concerned with the recovery experience of children who have been deeply injured by leukaemia, cancer and similar diseases, also shows us how social pathologies such as depression, anxiety and similar mental health epidemics of our present age could be formulated and better understood, and shows us how to approach the world differently in a situation imbued with social pathologies. This book reminds us of how important it is to have different languages and lenses to understand how contemporary society could evolve very differently from the pathogenic trajectory we are currently on: Peter Kearney shows us how we might turn things around.

Kieran Keohane
July 2018

Preamble

The preamble introduces my fascination with Serious Fun camps after see-ing their beneficial effects on children attending a leukaemia clinic, who had been subdued by treatment and then appeared transformed by a short holiday in Barretstown.

There has been very little historical writing about the camps, because Paul Newman did not wish to be centrepiece of any articles or publicity; rather he always hoped the focus would remain on the children and their camping experiences.

Howard "Doc" Pearson: *Founding Medical Director, Hole in the Wall Gang Camp*

In my latter years of paediatric practice that ranged from being a Leukae-mia Research Fellow in London to academic practice in Bristol and Cork, I naively assumed that the unexpected had disappeared from routine clinical challenges. I was aware of professional limits, and when faced with medical problems beyond my expertise, I usually knew who and where to consult and refer as necessary. There were still social issues that rankled and posed what seemed an insoluble quandary when trying to evaluate risks and ben-efits of advancing medical techniques and new treatments: what should be done when unavoidable side effects of new protocols seem to permanently undermine a child's spirit? A conventional answer suggested support from professionals in psycho-social departments, but the task seemed daunting and disheartening as the problem could not be resolved. The treatment protocols were lifesaving, but were also the root cause of the children's difficulties. Then, out of the blue, I was faced with an inexplicable and yet extraordinary transformation in seriously ill children who had attended the Irish Serious Fun camp in Barretstown, County Kildare. This book is to some extent the journey taken after observing that initial effect on children who had been on harsh treatments for cancer and leukaemia. There are many stories about the transforming effect of Serious Fun camps such as this heartfelt letter from a father whose son had attended camp:

During a ten-day period in Barretstown, kids can be happy and dis-connect from everything…you cannot imagine the positive change it has made to his life. Going to camp has opened to him a window to the world that was previously unknown to him. It was the first time he attended camp, the first time he went by himself without his family. We had tried several times before, but he never wanted to go. We did not insist too much as he was overprotected having a heart problem since he was very small. He always had problems to relate to others, he was very insecure, and faced every new situation with anxiety. Very slowly he was overcoming some of his fears until cancer appeared in his life. This made him go back with his self-confidence and although he faced the situation with a very mature attitude, he always showed himself sad and feeling lonely. When they talked to us about the possibility of going to Barretstown…his doctors encouraged us to send him…of course he did not want to go but finally…accepted. And as he now says, 'Thank God, I went, I have spent there the most happy ten days of my life'. He came back from camp totally renewed, feeling much more confident with himself, and most of all extremely happy. When we picked him up at the airport…he started telling us all about the camp; he was absolutely euphoric. He showed energy that we had not seen in him for a long time. He let all his emotions come out at Barretstown…I feel very emotional as I have seen my son happy.

There have been several psychological studies (Kiernan and McLaughlin, 2002; Kiernan et al., 2004; Meyler et al., 2010; Bekesi et al., 2011) that have sought to define the effect of Serious Fun camps in terms of self-esteem, resilience and quality of life, but they do not capture the sense of transformation reflected in that letter.

Sociology of health in twentieth-century Paediatrics

Medical advances in the twentieth century channelled practice towards increasing specialisation. In Paediatrics and Child Health, this demanded medical knowledge of disorders that interfere with physiological growth and social development of the child. Paediatric research focussed more on pathophysiology of childhood diseases than on repercussions of social experiences on children's health. Cultural blindness to health risks of social circumstances was unmasked to some extent by publication of Henry Kempe's famous article entitled 'The battered child syndrome' in 1962. Concealed parental violence was not routinely considered possible by health professionals up to then, but the public and the profession remained partially sighted as child sex abuse was still not admitted or recognised by health services until the 1980s. The importance of emotional context for children's health in hospital began to be acknowledged in the 1950s when an emphasis on hyperclean wards without parents shifted slowly to hospitals with child-friendly décor, play therapists and a nursing profession trained in the needs of children and their families; though toddlers fretting when separated from their families was common in children's wards up to the 1970s. Lonely toddlers rattled cot sides in baby wards until they 'settled'. This unintended social phenomenon of inconsolable fretting during early childhood was a travesty of hospital care, which only ceased when parents and carers were offered open access to their sick children. Misrecognition of these different kinds of child abuse as accidental rather than non-accidental injury, as non-specific medical complaints rather than symptoms of emotional abuse or fretting hospital behaviours as a psychological rather than a social pathology of separation anxiety must have been a nightmare for children. A happy family dream imagined by complacent governments and sanctimonious religions insulated society from these dark social realities. These examples of cultural blindness to the health risks of social circumstances are expressions of social pathology. The other side of the circumstantial coin – health benefits as a result of deliberate social interventions – are perhaps less well understood. These advantages were not the purpose of the first Serious Fun camp, the Hole in the Wall Gang Camp in Connecticut instituted by Paul Newman. His idea was that these children should be able to go to camp like their friends and siblings. The short holiday was simply intended as a respite and a break from the harsh treatment regimes of childhood cancer and leukaemia.

Child health statistics and the social dimension

Child health statistics reflect social conditions as well as medical causes of ill health, but at a more abstract population level than individual well-being. These figures are not alien to Paediatricians who are deeply aware of socio-economic factors impacting health measures. Child health morbidity and mortality figures have traditionally been socially stratified by parental employment and income levels. These statistics show significant health outcome differences ranging from social class one to five (Black et al., 1988). This social health gradient only measures physical health even though the gradient reflects both medical causes and stress-related mechanisms. However, health is a wider holistic concept that embraces both physical and spiritual dimensions to being alive. Valid and reliable statistics that measure morbidity and mortality throughout childhood have limitations as they do not account for the élan of living, perhaps the most important attribute of health (Nussbaum and Sen, 1993). New technologies drive changes in medical specialities, but exciting advances in molecular biology do not impact otherworldly dimensions to living. Quality of life and happiness studies fill this caring research vacuum, but their conclusions often seem trivial statements of the obvious (Schou and Hewison, 1999).[1]

Researching the social

Forty years of practice and perusal of the latest research in Paediatrics did not offer any assistance in understanding the transformation of sick children who had attended Barretstown, which seemed to be just a holiday camp. Most colleagues near retirement take to golf or resting with family and the next generation. It is usually a time for reflection whilst disengaging from the absorbing demands of hospital practice. The next generation of Paediatricians are in charge and you wish them bon voyage. There may be regrets, but the predominant feeling is of relief that the challenging anxieties of Paediatric practice are passing on to younger shoulders. However, curiosity about a transformation in seriously ill children prevailed and I took an opportunity to visit Barretstown in 2003. A year later I started reading Sociology in University College Cork. I retired from hospital practice in 2006, though I continued as a volunteer Paediatrician to Barretstown on an annual basis for a week or two until 2012. I travelled to the USA as a Visiting Scholar to the University of California, Berkeley, in 2008, and at the same time I could stay in the Painted Turtle Camp near Los Angeles as a researcher from Berkeley. I also visited the original Serious Fun camp – the Hole in the Wall Gang Camp in Connecticut – and could interview key informants there. I was a member of the Child Advisory Committee in Barretstown for several years. In 2010, I was a member of the Serious Fun Association's criterion assessment team that visited L'Envol French camp near Paris, the Over the Wall Gang Camp in the UK and the following year the Jordan River Valley camp in Israel. In 2011, I participated in volunteer training in Barretstown. I travelled to Moscow in 2012, where a Russian philanthropist was planning a new camp for seriously ill children along the lines of Serious Fun camps under the guidance of Terry Dignan, former Program Director in Barretstown. In 2016, I hoped to meet and interview Howard Pearson, the first medical director of the Hole in the Wall Camp, but sadly he passed away before my visit. There was compensation as I could interview Jimmy Canton and Bruce Maher. Jimmy had been in the Connecticut camp from the beginning and is currently CEO of the Hole in the Wall Gang Camp. Bruce is CEO of the Serious Fun Association. These multi-faceted experiences enriched my gradual understanding of Serious Fun camps, which I slowly realised had to be a social process of some kind. Sociology in Cork led by Professor Arpad Szakolczai and Dr Kieran Keohane was a fortuitous choice as the theoretical approach advocated there was as much from Anthropology as Sociology. As it turned out, their rich seam of Anthropologically grounded sociological theories and concepts was a crucial inspiration in my efforts to elucidate the extraordinary effectiveness of Serious Fun camps in promoting the welfare of seriously ill children.

Book title and subtitle

Salutogenesis literally means the origin of health and is a term introduced by Aaron Antonovsky (1979) to account for his research findings of seemingly inexplicable good health and *joie de vivre* in some survivors of the Holocaust. These survivors had been exposed to the most horrendous experience, but also had a prior 'sense of coherence' to their lives, which gave them extraordinary resilience and life-force. Salutogenesis is the counterweight to the more familiar term of pathogenesis – the causes of disease. Salutogenic experiences in Serious Fun camps for children with life-threatening illnesses may generate a social life-force with a holistic orientation to the world that parries our inevitable entropic doom.

The 'Butterfly' is taken from Jean Dominique Bauby's autopathography[2] 'The Diving Bell and the Butterfly' (2008), which has been made into a moving film of the same name. Bauby developed a catastrophic stroke aged forty-three while a very successful editor of 'Elle', a Parisian fashion magazine. He suffered from 'Locked in Syndrome', which is a condition of profound paralysis while retaining consciousness. The metaphor of a diving bell for his paralytic constraint was countered by a butterfly life-force that enabled Bauby to write the book through an alphabet of blinking signals devised by his imaginative speech therapist. The social constraints of illness can be lifted by liberating the butterfly within. The butterfly recurs in this book as a metaphor for venturesome living that embraces social health and well-being. It corresponds to Antonovsky's recognition of heterostasis as the underlying spirit of salutogenesis. The seeking butterfly of heterostasis contrasts with the steady state of homeostasis, the underlying physiological mechanism that maintains the status quo of physical health measures within a narrow range of normality.

Notes

1 Schou and Hewison complain that psychological aspects in quality-of-life measures in cancer care are still conceptualised in terms of physical function and fail to take account of the social experiences of treatment. They object to the fact that 'the bounded entity of the individual, separated from social context, is the focus of study'. They note the gap between the sophistication of statistical analysis and a weak conceptual grasp about quality of life.

2 An autopathography is the patient's tale (Aronson, 2006).

Introduction

Diagnoses such as childhood cancer trigger a process of social drama that persists during protracted treatments and the uncertainty of cure. Paediatricians considered Paul Newman's intuition about possible benefits of fun camps as an unnecessary risk for children with life threatening illnesses. Chapter 1 summarises the rapid progress in Paediatric Oncology as the context for the emergence of Serious Fun camps. Camp experiences outlined in chapter 2 entail radical separation of seriously ill children from home and hospital. Chapters 3 and 4 dissect different elements of health which can be impacted by camp. The Rite of Passage structure of camp discussed in chapter 5 assists healing when coupled to mimesis of trained mentors elaborated in chapters 6 and 7. Chapter 8 draws attention to inspirational leaders responsible for these major paradigm shifts in Paediatric care. Chapters 9 and 10 trace the spirit of Serious Fun camps from the emergence of American Summer Camps in the nineteenth century to its recent remarkable spread throughout the world. The conclusion summarises salutogenesis as a process facilitated by mimesis of exemplary mentors in a rite of passage.

> Once I lived like the Gods, and more is not needed.
>
> Hölderlin: *To the Fates*

This book is about special experiences (once I lived like the Gods), and how special experiences can shape our alignment with the world. The preamble outlines my obsession with trying to understand the benefits of Serious Fun camps, which do not make much sense from the perspective of medical science. Many of the best innovations are accidental findings and that seems to have been the case in the first Serious Fun camp founded by Paul Newman in 1988 that he called the Hole in the Wall Gang Camp. The original camp was simply meant to be a place of respite from hospitals for children with cancer and leukaemia, so that they could go to camp like their siblings and friends. Paul Newman's idea was that it should be a special refuge and hideout, where sick children could 'raise a little hell' (Pearson and Shefsky, 2016). It turned out to be much more than a break from hospital routines: a short time in the Hole in the Wall Gang Camp in Connecticut proved to be a pivotal life experience for these children with potentially fatal conditions. This was incomprehensible to me as a Paediatrician well versed in the pathophysiology of childhood disorders, but profoundly sceptical of words like magic and wonderland.

I seek to understand why Serious Fun camps happened when they did – in Weber's terminology – their conditions of emergence: what were the driving circumstances that led to the foundation of these special camps? Unique conditions of emergence set values that underpin the style and atmosphere of new institutions into the future (Szakolczai, 2003a), but first there must be a crisis that upsets the status quo – in this case a family emergency – that encourages new social formations. A life-threatening diagnosis such as acute leukaemia in children is a predicament that completely disrupts families from their everyday routines. The terrible threat of acute leukaemia and cancer in children eventually led to the emergence of Paediatric Oncology as a new subspecialty. The life-threatening prognosis of childhood malignancies changed from being almost uniformly fatal in the 1950s to a much better outlook. By the turn of the century, nearly nine out of ten children survived after treatment. Cancer survival is a partial triumph as the impact of treatment on survivors and non-survivors is still a largely untold story. Childhood cancer and leukaemia are unique conditions as they are relentlessly progressive, and the child will die in a matter of weeks or months if left untreated. Cancer treatment is a kind of necessary evil that must be tolerated for the greater good of survival. That is the crux of the problem. How can side effects of toxic drugs and inevitable social disruptions related to cancer treatment be ameliorated?

This book uses sociological concepts grounded in anthropology to provide a framework for understanding how these camps make a positive impact on sick children in such a short time. These concepts and social processes help clarify how peak experiences in special circumstance are central to experiential healing of children with life-threatening conditions. Liminality was the key concept that for me unlocked the mystery of social transformations in Serious Fun camps. Liminal conditions in a rite of passage structure relax social norms and provide challenging moments of danger as well as opportunity for change. The mantra of 'Challenge', 'Success', 'Reflection' and 'Discovery' adopted by European camps from the discipline of Therapeutic Recreation summarises the liminal process of Serious Fun transformation (Kearney, 2009). In terms of Anthropology, the process requires the presence of Masters of Ceremonies. Masters of Ceremonies are adepts, who in the context of Serious Fun camps are the Caras and Counselors that serve as guides and role models to the children, but they cannot be adepts without special training. Each camp has their own formal training process for their Caras or Counselors.[1]

The opening chapter outlines the development of new treatments for childhood cancer and leukaemia in the latter half of the twentieth century. Paediatric Oncology emerged from its first faltering experimental steps in the 1950s to its current position as one of the most demanding and exciting specialties in Paediatrics. Cancer treatments are harsh with serious side effects, so the focus of care needs attention to well-being as well as survival of the child. Most treatments are complete in a couple of years apart from a minority of resistant cases, which require very challenging interventions. The thrust for survival may trump social consequences and the specialty was slow to learn the skills of palliative care (Wolfe et al., 2000). An attempt is made to understand social difficulties that these children may face when their treatment is complete. As a young Paediatrician I was a participant and witness to both the hope and heartbreak of new protocols in the treatment of childhood leukaemia. From 1970, the Medical Research Council (MRC) saw the necessity for clinical research trials in children's leukaemia that could confirm in the UK reports of cures coming from the USA (Hardisty et al., 1981). In those days, Leukaemia Research Fellows worked as Paediatricians in the executive arms of MRC trials from UKALL I (United Kingdom Acute Lymphoblastic Leukaemia trial 1) to UKALL II and so on. Combination chemotherapy was a new approach in children. The sophisticated panoply of resources available to contemporary units of Paediatric Oncology in terms of pharmacy, anaesthesia, medical technology, specialist nurses and psycho–social support were not yet in place. The deep well of experience that guides clinical decisions was not available as procedures were novel and challenging. It was exhilarating and shocking as some children survived and others died (Kearney, 1976). The whole focus of treatment was on survival until survival became the rule rather than the exception. The clinical trial perspective gradually changed from a priority of cure to include concerns about quality of life in child cancer survivors (Eiser and Jenney, 2007). The social drama of diagnosis has consequences, and whilst traditional health support systems may alleviate economic issues and other hardships, the problem of unavoidable social exclusion during treatment cannot be resolved and may have long–term effects. The intensity of care took its toll on the social life of survivors interpreted here as a kind of Royal Stigma, an elaboration on Goffman's attribute of stigma (Goffman, 1990). The children are treated with great respect but at arm's length from society. I did not become aware of the liberating effect of Serious Fun experiences from the estrangement of Royal Stigma until thirty years after working as a Paediatrician in the MRC UKALL trials.

American summer camps such as the Hole in the Wall Gang Camp in Connecticut have turned out to be important interventions for children with life–threatening illnesses. These camps have developed from being an exclusive experience for elite young men in the latter half of the nineteenth century to more inclusive applications in the twentieth century. The prospect of curing children with cancer and leukaemia was the medical context for the development of Serious Fun camps. Paul Newman and Howard Pearson set a trajectory on how these new institutions should operate into the future with a focus on being child centred, playful, free of therapists and safe (Carlson and Cook, 2007). That approach has been retained in all Serious Fun camps, but that style of care does not reveal how or why these camps have such an impact on children with life–threatening conditions. Somehow the founders of Serious Fun camp experiences stumbled on social processes that profoundly affected the children's *joie de vivre*.

Chapter 2 emphasises the children's separation from their everyday routines during Serious Fun experiences. The children's feeling for camp is often described as magical. Magic implies a process beyond comprehension, but an outcome of the experience can be elaborated as post effervescent harmonic order, which can be understood as the opposite to post-traumatic stress disorder. It suggests how a short camping holiday could be a pivotal experience in the recovery of seriously ill children.

The next two chapters raise the question of health as a holistic term that embraces both physical and social health. The medical paradigm of health outlined in Chapter 3 materialises as a therapeutic response to pathogenesis. In contrast, the concept of salutogenesis in Chapter 4 takes a more holistic and inclusive perspective of health. These notions are outlined separately to tease out the distinction whilst recognising that physical and social health are intimately intertwined in practice. Medical interventions cope with pathogenesis – the causes of disease, whereas our social health requires salutogenesis[2] – the informing process of acquiring a healthy orientation to living.

Rites of passage are well recognised in common parlance as ritual processes that signify change in social status such the Bar Mitzvah when youths become adults or the crowning of monarchs. Chapter 5 suggests how the spatial and temporal structures around rites of passage may facilitate more than a change in social status. Healing rituals were disparaged by the Enlightenment as ridiculous magic, but censures by the scientific revolution need to be reconsidered. The magic can be translated into a more comprehensible narrative from the domain of social science. Rites of passage can be analysed and broken down into rites of separation from 'the real world', rites of transformation in liminal situations and rites of re-integration back into society. These rites can be variably recognised in the different camps. Feelings of camaraderie towards fellow campers and a sense of opportunity for change distinguishes the liminal space. Challenging experiences in a cohort of seriously ill children guided by specially trained carers can foster a salutogenic conversion of world view towards re-engagement with life and shedding of stigma. The final rite of re-integration restores newly ordered and healthful children back to society.

Chapter 6 tries to understand how a re-orientation of sick children can be achieved in such a short time. Interviews with alumni from Barretstown and the Painted Turtle pinpoint their relationships with Caras and Counselors during camp as the instrumental force for their change in attitude. Caras and Counselors are both Role Models and Masters of Ceremonies. Masters of Ceremonies need to be adept supervisors, and this requires formal training which Caras and Counselors undergo before camp. The mimetic process of subconscious imitation, long fostered by René Girard (1977) as the medium for subconscious desires that lead to rivalry and violence, can have an alternative beneficial impact on vulnerable children. Chapter 7 explores the mimetic apparatus of desire and how it may be the key to understanding how rites of separation, transition and re-integration are effective in transforming the attitude of sick children towards salutogenesis and recovery in such a short time.

Chapter 8 recounts the biographies of three twentieth-century prophets of paediatric care who with courage and daring overcame naysayers and imagined radical improvements in the medical and social management of children with cancer and leukaemia. Their vision came to pass in the institutions of St. Jude's Children's Research Hospital founded in 1962 and the Hole in the Wall Gang Camp that opened in 1988.

Chapter 9 identifies the emergence of Serious Fun camps from the institution of American summer camps. The camps originated in the middle of the nineteenth century for the reinvigoration of elite young Protestant men. These youths, when compared to their frontier forefathers, were seen as effete young fellows because of their pampered lifestyle due to industrialisation and urbanisation in the Northeastern United States. The camp approach was later adopted in Europe for good and ill by the Boy Scouts and Hitler Youth. In the USA, the summer camp experience became more democratic and, in the latter half of the twentieth century, began to adopt specific educational and therapeutic programmes. Chapter 10 recognises that Serious Fun camps have kept evolving and are now an international organisation of great repute.

The conclusion ties together the framework of a healing rite of passage and the mimetic process of salutogenesis, unwittingly adopted by Paul Newman to effect social transformations of severely ill children in Serious Fun camps. Serious Fun camps are oases of mimetic transformation in an era of social pathology. The ambition of the Series on the *Social Pathologies of Contemporary Civilization* is a more complete understanding of the collective *esprit de corps* in terms of our prevailing problems of health and well-being (Keohane et al., 2017). This book claims a place in the series as a small-scale response to Social Pathologies of Contemporary Civilization. Childhood cancer and leukaemia are not social pathologies, but the social implications of diagnosis and treatment can be substantial. The book suggests that individual psycho-social interventions are less effective than the special social experiences of Serious Fun camps. The camps provide a ready-made social process of transformation towards well-being. We stumble on social processes, which are then adopted by cultures after communal recognition of their power to govern change. The only social processes that transcend local cultures and become universal are those linked to survival and flourishing of the species like rites of passage and the sacrificial mechanism. Theorists confined imitation to the kindergarten in the twentieth century. The power of mimetic transformations remained masked by the suffix genesis as in psychogenesis, sociogenesis and salutogenesis. Genesis implies evolution, the gene and genetics and not Lamarck's inheritance of acquired characteristics. Then Girard rediscovered the pre-eminence of mimesis through literary scholarship. Caras and Counselors are Masters of Ceremonies and the prototypes for mimetic transformation. They weave the magic of the American Camp experience summarised in Europe by Therapeutic Recreation. Salutogenesis in healing rites of passage is a revolution in child care on par with the medical breakthroughs of Paediatric Oncology in the latter half of the twentieth century.

Notes

1 The Institute of Child Education and Psychology Europe (www.icepe.eu) and Thrive (www.thrive.ie) together with Trinity Consultants, Dublin, have offered specialised training for organisations, staff and volunteers working with children with additional needs (Dolan and Brady, 2011).
2 Salutogenesis as a concept has been adopted widely in Scandinavia and to a lesser extent by the rest of Europe. The Handbook of Salutogenesis (Mittelmark et al., 2017) has been published by Springer with open access online from www.springer.com/gp/book/9783319045993

1 Hope and heartbreak in Paediatric Oncology

The experimental nature of cancer chemotherapy trials in children drew criticism from Paediatricians sixty years ago, but their misgivings were matched by parents' desperation for a cure. It took twenty years before the specialty of Paediatric Oncology learned how to use cancer chemotherapy effectively; though not without a great deal of suffering for many children and their families in the interim. Childhood cancer survivors may have to cope with the effects of treatment on healthy tissue even when cured. Less well understood was survivors' conservative lifestyle. Their tentative participation in life can be understood as a manifestation of 'royal stigma'. Serious Fun camps in contrast were 'stigma free zones', where sick children could fully participate in available activities. The Hole in the Wall Gang Camp in Connecticut opened in 1988 and was simply intended as respite from hospital experiences but it proved to have unexpected beneficial consequences.

Primum non nocere

Hippocrates

After World War II, the new specialty of Paediatric Oncology introduced both hope and heartbreak to families who had children with conditions that up to then had been uniformly fatal. Hope was for children who might be cured, and heartbreak was for treatment failures, and sometimes even survivors whose care exacted a price of side effects both during treatment and long after the exacting challenges of therapy had been met. Immediate and long-term physical consequences of cancer treatments are well known (Oeffinger et al., 2006), but experiences of serious illnesses during childhood also have the potential to undermine well-being in survivors who – even as 'healthy' adults – may not 'flourish'. Increasing rates of 'surviving but not flourishing' emerge as a new kind of problem that can be understood in the historical context of therapeutic advances in childhood cancer and leukaemia. The breakthrough in cancer chemotherapy was dramatic and happened in children first. Fifty years ago, a diagnosis of childhood leukaemia was virtually a 'death sentence' whereas today survival rates are typically well over 80%.

Experiments

The extraordinary success of pharmacological drugs after World War II in treating infections led to a search for cancer chemotherapy. Old medical textbooks reveal the inadequacy of clinical medicine without antibiotics: gangrene, cavernous ulcers, abscesses and consumption – the old name for tuberculosis. So one can easily imagine the euphoria when the magic of antibiotics eradicated these conditions. It is not surprising that therapists saw cancer as their next target. The breakthrough in cancer chemotherapy was a slow drama. Researchers and therapists discovered drugs that had a temporary effect against acute leukaemia in children. In 1948, Sydney Farber and colleagues from the Boston Children's Medical Centre published results of experimental chemotherapy (Farber et al., 1948). The article was about remission and relapse of acute leukaemia in children. At first, the drugs produced what seemed to be a miraculous remission – the disease disappeared from the perspective of available measures. Then the leukaemia relapsed and the children died. It took another twenty years before these experimental drugs were sufficiently understood to make a breakthrough to cure.

Effective anti-cancer drugs happened first in Paediatric Oncology. This was a surprise as a generally accepted unwritten rule of human research was that new treatments should be tried in adults first. Some Paediatricians were unhappy with experimental cancer chemotherapy in children especially when new problems arose because of severe side effects. Needle phobia, isolation and the unwanted consequences of chemotherapy were extremely difficult for children, their families and hospital staff responsible for their care. A colleague of Sydney Farber noted an ethical dimension against these treatments summarised by a catch phrase 'Let them die in peace' (Mercer, 1999). The initial flurry of excitement due to temporary remissions abated. The profession regarded Farber's clinical research as experimental and not a breakthrough. Paediatricians reverted to their contention that trials of new drugs should not be tested on children first, and when asked recommended supportive care only to parents of children with malignancies. Discussions with families were confined to whether comfort was enhanced by blood transfusions, and that remained the case in most centres until the 1960s and 1970s.

Therapeutic turn in Paediatrics

In or about 1970, the discipline of Paediatrics changed. The change was not sudden and definite. But a change there was, nevertheless; and, since one must be arbitrary, let us date it about the year 1970.[1] You could say that up to then the possibility of fatal infectious disorders dominated Paediatrics. After World War II, new antibiotics, immunisations and better standards of living gradually overcame the threat of dangerous infections. For most of the twentieth-century childhood cancers and leukaemia were a footnote to the practice of Paediatrics, but around 1970 these disorders acquired a new visibility. The prevalence of childhood cancers increased year upon year as some children survived, whereas formerly they only lived a few weeks or months after diagnosis. Annual figures for incidence and prevalence of childhood cancer were the same when these malignancies were rapidly lethal. Towards the millennium, the prevalence of childhood cancer survivors increased as more and more children responded to new treatment protocols. Smith et al. (2010) reported a decline in childhood cancer mortality rates by more than 50% between 1975 and 2006. They also noted an unexplained increase in the incidence rates of childhood cancer that was most pronounced for acute lymphoblastic leukaemia. This new visibility of childhood cancer and leukaemia had a striking appearance. Affected children during therapy looked like medical waifs – as if they had been neglected. They lost hair, lost weight and failed to thrive, so their suffering was apparent with almost shades of the Shoah. They became headline news as it dawned on the public that cancer could occur in children as well as adults. Paediatric medicine changed. The main emphasis in Children's Hospitals was no longer about treatment of acute infectious disorders. The lethal threat of meningitis, epiglottitis and septicaemic shock gradually waned. The main remit of Paediatric services shifted from urgent treatment of acute infections to protracted engagement with complex chronic disorders. Innovative treatments and technologies were now able to alleviate chronic severe life-threatening conditions with childhood cancer and leukaemia as prime examples.

History of a breakthrough in cancer chemotherapy

Paediatric Pathologists and Haematologists in the early twentieth century confined their research to morphological classifications of different types of childhood cancers and leukaemia. These distinctions assisted clinicians in making a prognosis and determining whether there was a possibility of cure through surgery and radiotherapy. Histology revealed the crucial distinction of whether tumours were benign or malignant. The former could be cured but the prognosis for malignancies was bleak. Childhood malignancies are different from adult cancers as they mainly occur in connective tissues derived from mesoderm – embryonic cells in between external ectoderm and internal endoderm. Ectoderm and endoderm mature into surface tissues of skin and internal tracts. They are the source of common adult cancers in the gut and skin. Childhood malignancies are also demarcated from adult cancers by their speed of growth leading to a devastating short duration between onset and death if left untreated. Cancers in adults have a more insidious onset and lengthy course that results in a slower demise if surgery and radiotherapy are ineffective.

Ancient and modern medicine

History credits Hippocrates with the axiom 'to cure sometimes, relieve often and comfort always'. Modernity in the sense of a scientific approach to medical remedies did not intrude on clinical therapeutics until after World War II. Before then textbooks of Materia Medica, the pharmacopoeias of effective treatments, accumulated expertise over centuries through experience. Materia Medica textbooks were organised by the alphabet rather than based on an understanding of how these drugs worked: A for atropine, B for bismuth, C for calcium, D for digitalis and so on. The ambition of Physicians and their Materia Medica was modest and complied with the Hippocratic axiom 'to cure sometimes' until well into the twentieth century. The discovery of penicillin, sulphonamides and the needs of war stimulated research into new drugs. The burgeoning specialty of Clinical Pharmacology had a strong biochemical foundation. This more scientific and effective approach replaced Materia Medica as the therapeutic discipline for medical students and the profession. Pharmaceutical research moved from academia in university hospitals to become a thriving industry in multi-national locations. The old order of the Hippocratic axiom shifted so that initial expectations of medical interventions became 'to cure often'. 'To comfort always' was now hardly needed as antibiotics were quickly effective against infections that were formerly life threatening. Cancer chemotherapy was different. These drugs were toxic to both healthy and malignant tissues. The Hippocratic axiom had to adjust again if cancer chemotherapy was going to be sanctioned for treatment. *Primum non nocere* – first do no harm – the reproach from medical ethics had to be shelved. *Primum nocere* became necessary if childhood cancer was going to be treated. The administration of cancer chemotherapy necessitated downgrading the comfort injunction as harm was unavoidable. 'To comfort always' became unrealistic as physical and psycho–social consequences of treatment were unrelenting. For parents, the consequences had to be endured as the alternative was the death of their child.

Emergence of Paediatric Oncology

Sydney Farber's contribution to treating acute leukaemia in children was not forgotten. He had clearly shown that certain drugs had a transient beneficial effect against acute leukaemia, but physical and social costs of a temporary chemotherapy remission were too demanding to become an acceptable standard approach for mainstream practice. Sydney Farber was a Paediatric Pathologist of international renown and regarded as the founder of cancer chemotherapy, but he did not make the crucial breakthrough in childhood acute leukaemia. In the 1950s, childhood cancer had a kind of a heroic visibility in the USA through fundraising publicity such as the 'Jimmy Fund' (Krueger, 2007). Fundraising was very successful, and led to new clinics for children with cancer, but the prognosis did not change. Farber's programme of sequentially testing new single-agent chemotherapy did not improve the long-term outlook until Frei and Freireich introduced the concept of combination chemotherapy (Frei III et al., 1958, 1961). These Clinical Cancer Investigators were stalwarts of research and there may not have been a breakthrough in chemotherapy without them; but the downside was relentless ambition for a cure at the expense of dying children. At the National Cancer Institute, Bethesda, the children's leukaemia ward began to be called a 'butcher shop' (Mukherjee, 2010). Combination chemotherapy entailed using as many as four drugs together to get around the problem of drug resistance, which had thwarted Farber's earlier attempts at finding a cure through escalating doses of single drugs. In single-agent chemotherapy, the drug dose was pushed to the limit of toxicity. Drugs used in combination had different side effects and when used in lower doses together were less toxic than single-agent chemotherapy pushed to the limit of tolerance. Longer remissions were achieved but the leukaemia relapsed in the central nervous system. The crucial breakthrough came after the establishment of St. Jude's Children's Research Hospital in Memphis, Tennessee, where clinical trials led by Donald Pinkel and his team throughout the 1960s resulted in the first reliable cures of acute lymphoblastic leukaemia (Rivera et al., 1993).

Heartbreak

'The Child First and Always' was a logo on the lintel over the old entrance to the Hospital for Sick Children, London, that expressed an ideal of best practice for Paediatricians. This ideal did not suit many of those researchers for whom a cure for cancer was a kind of obsession fortified by desperate parents. These clinicians were not well versed in the skills of palliative care and often pursued aggressive chemotherapy until the child died. By the year 2000, three out of four children were cured of their cancer in the USA, but there was a price to be paid by those whose treatment was unsuccessful. Wolfe et al. (2000) reported from a centre of excellence that children resistant to standard chemotherapy still received aggressive treatment at the end of life. Nine out of ten of these children suffered 'a lot or a great deal' from at least one symptom in their last month of life. The authors recommended that greater attention must be paid to palliative care for children who are dying of cancer. A similar report from Australia ten years later (Heath et al., 2010) revealed more home deaths and fewer unsuccessful medical interventions, suggesting a more realistic approach to end of life care for Australian children dying of cancer.

Childhood cancer survivors

Cancer and leukaemia are still the epitome of life-threatening illnesses in children even though the prognosis has vastly improved. Survival rates have changed dramatically so that long-term survival in childhood cancer is now over 80% (Hewitt et al., 2003). The treatment is harsh and even in the best of hands the children's health-related quality of life is significantly poorer than their healthy peers (Eiser, 2004). They miss out on full-time education and experience problems on returning to school (Larcombe et al., 1990). There have been reports of post-traumatic stress and similar disorders in a small minority of survivors (Langeveld et al., 2004). As adults, their lifestyle is remarkably conservative. They are less likely than their contemporaries to be smokers, drink alcohol or use recreational drugs (Larcombe et al., 2002). A more detailed study about the course of life in survivors of childhood cancer confirmed that survivors showed less risk-taking behaviour than their peers (Stam et al., 2005). Their education was on par with their peers, but they married less often and were more frequently unemployed. The evidence suggests that the consequences of childhood cancer and leukaemia are not over after completing treatment (Gurney et al., 2009). The physical side effects of the different treatments can be monitored and treated, but the social effects of childhood cancer and its treatment may be more insidious and disabling as they can sideline survivors from full participation in life, perhaps best summarised by the attribute of stigma.

Royal Stigma

The stigma of chronic severe illness in children is unusual because these children are generally treated with great sympathy and sometimes pity. This has the paradoxical effect of making matters worse by separating these vulnerable children from their peers. It is a kind of Royal Stigma as the children are treated with great respect and concern but are isolated from the hurly burly of life. According to Goffman (1990), stigma is an individual's situation when he is disqualified from full social acceptance. It is an elusive term as parameters of social acceptance vary with time and place.

Etymology of stigma

Stigma singles out individuals from the crowd and focusses communal attention on attributes of distinction or shame:

> That snotty urchin
> Left unpicked
> by either team...
> Ah the bitter cold!
>
> SHIKI

The etymology of stigma can be traced to ancient Greece, where the term originated as a tattoo mark of distinction for those in service of the temple (Whitehead et al., 2001). This branding with a hot iron was later used as a method to identify slaves and criminals. The process was the same, but the social significance of the stigmatic tattoo had changed from a sign of distinction to a mark of shame. In the Christian era, stigmata were believed to be a bodily sign of holy grace as they expressed identification with Christ's suffering. In Ophthalmology, a diagnosis of astigmatism, implying an absence of stigmatism, is a common cause of blurred vision: a distorted lens impairs the focussing power of the eye. These apparent differences in meaning can be reconciled by recognising stigmatism as a communal process of attentive focus on attributes that are unusual – sufficiently rare in statistical terms to be a couple of deviations above or below the norm. Individuals in all communities have a propensity to gradually separate into layers of distinction. The normal majority have attributes that are acceptable to one another reflecting prevailing communal values. Their different beliefs are tolerable as they do not trouble other members of the group. The prevailing values of the majority do not command focussed attention. They are astigmatic to one another as they do not have values and beliefs, which clearly mark them as separate from their community. Stigmatisation occurs when minorities deemed to have exceptional vices or virtues are subject to attentive scrutiny by the majority. Goffman states that stigma is an attribute that is deeply discrediting, but that is not the way in Christian stigmata, which are a sign of holy grace. Stigmatisation is more a communal perspective that recognises deviance from the norm, but not necessarily discrediting as exceptional deviance can be a sign of graceful distinction as well as shameful disgrace. Stigma may apply to royalty as well as outcasts, but there is another twist to this mercurial trait. Stigma can disappear. There are situations where stigma may not apply. Goffman refers to some people who are 'wise' with a wide range of social values that can include deviants from the norm. Children with disability may be stigmatised at school but cherished and loved at home. Stigma is not a permanent slur as 'the wise' can create stigma-free zones, where viewpoints embrace difference. Stigma can then be reconciled in different areas and eras as an endpoint of a social process that focusses on attributes recognised as exceptional or deplorable by the prevailing zeitgeist.

The end of stigma?

There are times when stigma can be shaken and reformed even to the extent that Gill Green suggests the possible end of stigma due to changes in social experiences of long-term illness (Green, 2009). The target of stigmatisation due to health issues has shifted within living memory, from TB to Cancer to AIDS to dementia as these former unmentionables fraught with risk and suffering became less demonised. The end of stigma seems a premature judgment of innate human tendencies to distinguish 'the other' as different. Stigmas of race, religion and migrants are still at the forefront of politics. The stigmatised person can be made a scapegoat – an innocent bystander – whose non-participation in prevailing social values renders them vulnerable to arbitrary victimisation. A scapegoat is the clearest example of marginalisation, but most kinds of social exclusion are less obvious and more subtle and discreet.

Stigma is an individual's situation when disqualified from full social acceptance (Goffman, 1990). Uncertainty of status for the stigmatised person operates in a wide variety of social situations. The visibly stigmatised individual will feel anxious due to unanchored interaction in mixed social situations. In stigma theory, attributes are imputed from appearances. Stigmatised persons become aware of sympathetic others who do not share prevailing prejudices. These may be because of a stigma shared or because they are 'wise'. Goffman describes a stigma shared as something that may begin with a shudder but ends up as freemasonry. A stigma shared may also be a turning point life event when an individual learns that fully fledged members of the group are quite like ordinary human beings. The wise are usually either a member of family or a professional expert. In Serious Fun camps, there is full social acceptance of manifold appearances, so that exceptional health issues become the norm. The prevailing wisdom there is of tolerance and encouragement in a stigma-free zone.

Stigma-free zones

Serious Fun camp experiences can be one of the ways to shake up and reform stigma. They may reverse cultural effects of chronic severe childhood illnesses through pivotal social experiences that are recognised as great achievements by their peers and valued counselors. Part of camp benefit may be erasure of a personal social identity that is devalued in some social circumstances. Stigma is perhaps best understood as a cultural term. Culture is inherently unstable and subject to prevailing climates of opinion. One of the strengths of Serious Fun camps is a deliberate policy of being stigma-free zones. This can be sustained because of their complete separation from the 'real world'. Furthermore, the collective effervescence and communitas of camp discourages any emerging layers of social distinction. Human beings in groups will always sediment at different rates, but it takes time. A brief week in camp, even if it is an experience of a lifetime, is too short for the emergence of social distinctions.

There is a final ironic quirk in attribution of stigma. It can be confronted by the stigmatised. Stigma that is resisted may reverse the process as happened to Oscar Pistorius, who needed both his lower limbs amputated as an infant. He could have been stigmatised but his achievements as Blade Runner and Paralympian gold medallist made him a national hero in South Africa. In 2009, Gill Green chose his photograph as front piece for her book *The End of Stigma?*. The wheel of stigma turned again in 2013 when Pistorius was found guilty of shooting and killing his girlfriend, South African model Reeva Steenkamp. His emotional outbursts about his disability during the trial did not convince the court (Scheper-Hughes, 2014).

Morbidity, mortality and quality of life

The sudden threat of acute infectious disorders is no longer a major concern in the Western World. This changing prognosis in diseases of children from acute life-threatening infections to chronic complex disorders marked a therapeutic turn in Paediatrics. Improved survival rates in cancer and leukaemia shifted emphasis from mortality to issues related to the morbidity of the disease and its treatment. The focus of research in childhood malignancies is no longer just about surviving but now embraces the long-term well-being of survivors. Treatment protocols for childhood cancer and leukaemia may result in 'Royal Stigma' – a kind of revered social exclusion – that can impact on survivors' future well-being. As patients they typically experience separation and isolation from school, peers and family during protracted treatments. Even after treatment has completed they must live with the threat of relapse and long-term consequences of their chemotherapy and radiotherapy. Sixty years ago, the issue for children with cancer and leukaemia was the immediacy of death, and almost without exception their quantity of life after diagnosis was painfully short. Paediatric Oncologists had to be concerned about quality of life when survival became the rule rather than the exception. Quality-of-life issues around physical health can be documented reliably (Bhakta et al., 2017), but physical health is often subservient to circumstances related to stigma and its impact on social and emotional health. The stigma of chronic childhood illnesses is a relatively new phenomenon as it is directly related to improved treatments for children who would have died in former times. Protocols of cancer chemotherapy often inadvertently marginalise children from their families and class mates. Effective drugs for childhood cancer and leukaemia were available soon after World War II, but it took over twenty years for the profession to make a breakthrough to a reliable cure in St. Jude's Children's Hospital. It took much longer for Serious Fun camps to be recognised as an effective intervention for children inadvertently marginalised from their friends and families. The Hole in the Wall Gang Camp in Connecticut that opened in 1988 was the first Serious Fun camp for seriously ill children. It was intended as a respite for children with cancer and leukaemia from overwhelming hospital experiences, where they could for a short while 'raise a little hell'. Serious Fun experiences proved to be much more than respite from hospital protocols.

Note

1 Paraphrased from Virginia Woolf's essay – Mr Bennett and Mrs Brown – on change in 1910.

2　Serious Fun experiences

Chapter 2 emphasises the children's separation from their everyday routines during Serious Fun experiences. The children's feeling for camp is often described as magical. Magic implies a process beyond comprehension, but memorable consequences can be elaborated as post effervescent harmonic order – a sense of coherence – which can be understood as the opposite to post traumatic stress disorder. It implies that a short camping holiday could be a pivotal experience in the recovery of seriously ill children. This state has symptoms in common with post-traumatic stress disorder such as flashbacks and hyperarousal symptoms triggered by unforgettable circumstances, but they are on the opposite side of the memory coin: one is joyful, the other fearful.

> Imagination is the only weapon in the war against reality.
>
> Lewis Carroll: *Alice in Wonderland*

There is already a sense of disorientation in a journey to camp even before you arrive, as their locations are off the beaten track and hard to find. The Irish camp at Barretstown Castle is only forty miles from Dublin, but the entrance is situated in a network of byroads and it is easy to get lost. Parents complain about the lack of signposts. At the gate, you tap in a code or else you need to identify your credentials over the intercom. Then the gates slowly swing open, miming a gracious invitation to participate in a different world. The vista is pastoral and the drive sweeps past grazing sheep and horses with little indication that the castle is home to the Barretstown experience for seriously ill children. The gate closes automatically and excludes the 'real world'. At reception, you are given a name tab to remind fellow campers who you are, but identifications are confined to first names only, alerting everyone that worldly titles and status have no meaning in camp. Then it seems that everyone has known you forever as greetings become warm, friendly and open. In the castle grounds, there is a sense of quiet respect for everybody within the estate even though many of the social interactions are boisterous and unrestrained.

Separation from the real world

These first impressions of Barretstown had a curious unspoken mix of carnival and the sacred that seem to be a feature of all Serious Fun camps. The camps have an international presence in the twenty-first century that is an extraordinary expansion from the original Connecticut 'Hole in the Wall Gang Camp' founded by Paul Newman and Howard Pearson in 1988. The entrance to that camp in the small town of Ashford is low key, but the surprise of a beautiful campus may be augmented by the unreality of waves from passing cross-dressers.[1] It is the same sense of stepping into the unknown that pervades when sweeping up Castle Avenue in Barretstown. The Painted Turtle camp is only seventy miles north of Los Angeles, but it might as well be in another continent, as the design is of a remote African village. It is easily bypassed as it blends into the dry and arid landscape. The French camp L'Envol is in a chateau forty miles south of Paris, but even old hands find it difficult to find the entrance. Jordan River Valley, the camp in Israel, is easy to see from afar, but is difficult to know in the Middle Eastern glare whether it is real or a mirage like an oasis in the desert. The multilingual welcomes on the camp gates in Hebrew, Arabic and European languages are made surreal by whistling gale sounds from low flying F15 jets that suddenly disrupt the peace. Over the Wall camp in the UK has no permanent location, but all the camps have a magical dreamlike quality that on arrival disconnects participants from the real world.

The campers' isolation from the everyday is not just geographical but also social and psychological as they leave behind their worlds of hospital regimes and anxious families. Most camps establish a media-free location for the campers. All kinds of communication with the outside world are deliberately disconnected. There are no social media and all mobile phones must be handed in. There is no Internet, television, radio or newspaper for the campers. They are entirely dependent on one another for all kinds of gossip and information. Not all camps are perfect in this regard and there is some evidence that camps are less successful if they operate a more open policy of permitting campers to communicate with the outside world. That is a brief first impression of camp and it seemed to me a strange experience, as Europeans unlike Americans have not got a tradition of entrusting sick children to residential holiday camps during the summer.

Serious Fun

Serious Fun is almost an oxymoron, but it has been chosen as the name for the international organisation of holiday camps for seriously ill children. The association was originally called the Hole in the Wall Gang Association after the first camp. The camps spread to Ireland and then to all continents, but as the association grew the name was considered unwieldy. The association chose Serious Fun, the motto of Barretstown for the twenty-first century, as a suitable name to rebrand an organisation with international responsibilities. Serious achievements and poking fun summarise the ambitions of holiday camps for children with life-threatening illnesses. Serious achievements in playful activities reveal unsuspected abilities in ill children, whilst poking fun at conventions in general and those of medicine in particular are both integral parts of the experience.

Original aim of Serious Fun camps

Paul Newman's original aim was to provide a kind of temporary sanctuary for children from their hospital world where they could 'raise a little hell'. Newman's ambition was realised, but there was an unexpected beneficial consequence. The children were apparently transformed by their experience. The medical perspective was of no avail in understanding why a short holiday in a special camp for seriously ill children makes a real and long-term difference to the campers. According to their parents, family and health carers, sick children were changed for life by their experiences that had lasted only from five to ten days. There was nothing in the medical tomes that could enlighten a Paediatrician about what was happening. The Serious Fun Network is aware that the camp does much more than allow seriously ill children 'raise a little hell'. They recognise the transforming power of their camps and state that their programmes are purposefully designed to 'foster independence, resilience and personal growth, helping children to see beyond the limits of their medical conditions and experience all that life has to offer'.[2]

Magic

'Magic' was the standard answer to queries about why Barretstown seemed so effective in such a short time, but magic could not be formally investigated as Paul Newman, the founder of Serious Fun camps, placed an embargo on all kinds of research on children during the camp. His intuition was probably correct, as formal research interviews or surveys during the camp could have broken the spell of wonderland. A role as volunteer Paediatrician gave me a privileged observer position in the camp as I was a member of the medical staff and not a visiting researcher. I could interview senior administrative staff and they were very aware of Barretstown as a magical experience:

> The magic thing is, it sounds ridiculous, the way everyone says its magic or whatever, but it's so true. It is hard to describe but it is tangible. I still can't tell you what that magic is. Anybody that comes down and becomes part of it. They understand it straight away. There is real kind of cause behind what we do here. You can see with your own eyes, I mean what Barretstown does for these kids.

In Barretstown, there is a 'Harry Potter drawer' that harbours notes from parents:

> A father wrote from Scotland: Jimmy left us twelve days ago and we sent him to Ireland. He has not come back the same child.

Parents speak to staff with the same kind of story:

> She had a fantastic time and met some lovely people. She was brave enough to try canoeing and climbing. No mean task when you have only one leg and poor eyesight. I was particularly pleased that she had joined in with some dancing as she has not attempted this since she had her leg amputated so it was a particular triumph for her.

A former CEO of Barretstown was convinced of the effectiveness of the camp by talking to parents:

> My view tends to come more from talking to parents that their children weren't able to socialise and now they are. I was talking to one of the dads. I said what made you come here – that kind of thing. He said well I wanted to see what happened to my son who had come on a ten-day program. He was extremely clear about how before he came he wouldn't go to school, he never played out, he was very withdrawn, a computer nerdy type. And he said when he came back he was so different. He wanted to come and experience what his son had experienced.

Magical communitas

Serious Fun camps have an atmosphere that becomes apparent once the 'real world' has been excluded. It is a magical mood of friendliness that generates a sense of communitas between campers. Communitas was a term introduced by Victor Turner (1969) to distinguish exhilarating social relationships from mundane interactions in everyday life. For Turner, community was an area of common living, whereas communitas was a mode of special human relationships. He used the term for a style of communication amongst a young cohort undergoing traditional rites of passage in liminal situations overseen by benevolent Masters of Ceremonies. Communitas with its unstructured character represents the 'quick' of I–thou relations and involves the whole person in relation to the whole of other persons. In comparison, the structure of the 'real world' has a purely cognitive tone and is essentially a set of social categories. Wit and imagination are the hallmarks of communitas with a style of human interaction that may vary from humour, dance and discourse to drawing and stories, but with the recognition that they derive from fresh metaphor – those golden moments when layers of narrative interact with present discourse revealing dazzling new insights, intuitions and activities. These inspirational moments or durations may recast the previous structure in an innovative way. Magical communitas is a very different experience for the campers compared to the social structure of formal interactions with hospital treatment protocols and disciplinary health rules at home. In the camp, the focus is on children having fun as noted by a programme director:

> The focus is on the child having fun rather than on the illness; for the kids, its really very precious for them. And they don't mind coming out with loads of jargon because people understand it here. The kids will have a full-blown conversation about names of drugs that are about ten million words long. They are all yapping away and its totally fine to do that over the dinner table. And it's just that sense of belonging here. Because everybody understands and that's one of the biggest things for kids. That affirmation and feeling that they belong somewhere.

Group interviews with camp alumni as adults circumvented Newman's injunction against interviewing children during the camp. Many years after the camp, these Barretstown graduates fondly remembered their short time in the camp as a pivotal life experience. The social interaction amongst themselves as campers was memorable and evident to any casual observers of the camp:

> I remember my first day I came everyone was so friendly, everyone was on their own, you made friends straight away, getting to know people how exciting it was, the fun!

Relationships at home prior to camp were often fraught with anxiety:

> At home you were treated different, people were always worrying about you, it was like they were wrapping you in cotton wool, even brushing your teeth had people worrying…It was hard to adjust to life back home, here you were treated as an adult.

The magic of brilliant camp relationships with fellow campers and counselors transformed the anxious relationships at home:

> My ma was so surprised when I went home I started crying she said why are you crying? I wanted to go back. I wanted to live there, she laughed! I was telling her it was like a dream come true. We were all the same now, you didn't have to hide your feelings or hide who you were, you could just let loose meeting all those people… When I found out I had my illness, I felt alone I thought I was the only person in the world with the sickness, afraid to talk to people. My Mom never understood, there was always trouble, tension not trouble, emotions. As soon as I came here they understood. I was able to go home and say that what I have. I am not the only person who is sick. They understood then. I came away a totally different person.

And not only at home but also their tentative relationships with healthy friends:

> Before I came I found it was hard to make friends. With the illness, you go to talk about it they think it is a disease or something they don't want to hang around with you. Before I came I was quiet After coming here I got more confidence, I became more outspoken trying to talk to people about different things.

Relationships with the opposite sex could be problematic for a teenager with a serious illness:

> If you are in a club I was afraid to meet boyfriends or tell them in case they would run or something, if you tell someone they would say, what!? After I came here I got confidence, I don't care, they like you for who you are, if not – see you later.

Nobody was clear what the magic was, other than an almost tangible asset for engaging the world. Serious Fun magic seemed to be about changing relationships: about how campers related to themselves, to one another, to their families and to the world.

Collective effervescence

Aside from communitas of magical relationships between campers the experience itself has a quality of excitement perhaps best expressed by Durkheim's term of collective effervescence (Durkheim, 1995). This was very evident in the dining halls and the tearful time of departure. Some campers have experienced almost all aspects of Serious Fun institutions because they started as seriously ill campers for a few summer sessions before returning as volunteers, and finally, as paid members of staff. Such a camper who is now a qualified professional noted the irony that going home after the camp was for him a most stressful time:

> It is stressful. I think the most stressful time for me was going home that third time. The first time was horrible and hard, but I knew there was a possibility of coming back. And I got back. And that was OK. I got through that session again next time when I wanted to come back. I knew at that last summer, the end of the third one, I couldn't get back. I wasn't getting back. And that was more stressful than the first one. The second was fine like there wasn't anything stressful regards going home. The first time I went home I cried my eyes out, the whole way home because I wanted to go back. The second time, well it was calm, it was fun going home. The third time going home I was a lot quieter a lot more – OK, the reality is then I don't have that to go back to – No more Barretstown, but I do have what it gave me.

Barretstown had been a kind of external magical resource that could after a time be kept and become an internal resource to face the future. That Barretstown alumnus still gets spontaneous physiological reactions on return to Barretstown by a route that reprises his first visit to camp. He feels his heart thumping and gets flashbacks of his former experiences:

> It's got to the point where you drive in the front gate and you come around and see the castle, and your heart just goes nuts. You are shaking. You are sweating. And it's just fantastic…It's a feeling that brings me back every single time to that place where it was something different, something new, something special. It's a really good feeling, being here at all, brings back so many memories of being that it's OK to be different or that it's OK to be who you are. It was more a feeling inside, coming back each time. There was this kind of feeling inside when I came back that it just almost got giddy at getting here

Barretstown was a decisive change in his life. Before Barretstown, he led a very constrained life dominated by his illness. The long-term beneficial effects of Barretstown for him are real and permanent as they have been a pivotal life experience, completely changing his outlook and ambition:

> For me its lots of fun, because this is where I feel the safest. This is the place where I got a lot of ideas and a lot of my memories from childhood. I was doing some maths say from zero to fifteen years, the time I spent here is less than one per cent. I'd say that about fifty per cent of my best childhood memories are here. And that comparison, like I have some good memories from outside, but the best memories are from here from people; not specifically high ropes or archery or activities, but people, other kids and just being able to feel OK.

Post effervescent harmonic order

I call this Serious Fun effect 'post effervescent harmonic order' that settles inside after the excitement of collective effervescence and convivial communitas. This state has something in common with post-traumatic stress disorder with flashbacks and hyperarousal symptoms triggered by particular circumstances, but on the opposite side of the memory coin: one is joyful, the other fearful. The classical symptoms of post-traumatic stress disorder are re-experiencing symptoms, avoidance of reminders of trauma, symptoms of hyperarousal and emotional numbing occurring a variable time after a traumatic event (NICE, 2005). Post-traumatic stress disorder is classically associated with major trauma such as rape, war and catastrophic events. The condition is now a recognised consequence of life-threatening illnesses and has been reported as a rare complication of childhood cancer experiences (Taieb et al., 2003), though Langeveld et al. (2004) reported that some symptoms of post-traumatic stress disorder were present in 12% of survivors. Post effervescent harmonic order by contrast is a healthy process of reformed orientation to living and a renewed world view. It is in many ways, like the process of salutogenesis, a concept introduced by Antonovsky in 1979 to distinguish a neutral or beneficial consequence of stress from the standard view of stress as a cause of disease. Stress was invariably pathogenic in the medical literature of the time, but Antonovsky had an alternative perspective on stress with a paradoxical view that stress was not always pathogenic and could at times be healthful or salutogenic. Post effervescent harmonic order then is a consequence of salutogenic experiences – a recalibration of world views. It does not contain a moral stance but is rather a quiet confidence in personal abilities that can utilise available resources to face life's challenges. It is perhaps one way of achieving a version of Antonovsky's sense of coherence, the key concept of salutogenesis. For Antonovsky, a salutogenic sense of coherence is an apprehension that the world can be understood assisted by personal, social and cultural resources that reveal our participation in life's challenges as meaningful and worthwhile.

Children who attend Serious Fun camps have life-threatening illnesses and this medical aspect of their health needs to be clarified before appraising the role of salutogenesis as a satisfactory explanation of Serious Fun camping experiences. The medical and social dimensions to health are intimately linked but need to be separated in order to explicate their overlapping contributions to child health.

Notes

1 The fancy dress of Caras and Counselors often includes cross-dressing – evidence of their spontaneous undermining of categories from the real world that no longer apply in the magical world of Serious Fun.
2 (www.linkedin.com/company/seriousfun-children's-network/) accessed 29/11/17.

3 Mirage

The medical paradigm of health

It is necessary to separate medical health from quality of life whilst recognising that they are intimately related when trying to understand the beneficial consequences of Serious Fun camps. The Medical model of health is negative, like a mirage, as it represents an absence of disease. It is founded on the self-regulating mechanism of homeostasis that challenges pathogenesis and maintains physiological processes in a steady state. Children who attend Serious Fun camps are seriously ill and they are still seriously ill when they leave, and yet they are 'transformed', more healthful. An absence of pathogenesis does not guarantee health. For Antonovsky health was a positive force for living that he called salutogenesis, that in many circumstances was more important than various causes of pathogenesis and their associated deficits in homeostasis

> The core of the new doctrine was that each disease had a well-defined cause and that its control could best be achieved by attacking the causative agent or, if this was not possible, by focusing treatment on the affected part of the body. This was a far cry from the emphasis placed by ancient medicine on the patient, and on his total environment.
>
> René Dubos: *Mirage of Health*

René Dubos (1959/1988) as a distinguished microbiologist recognised perhaps better than most that the new doctrine of specific aetiology espoused by Pasteur and Koch in the nineteenth century was a powerful but insufficient explanation of how disease disrupts health. Searching for a specific aetiology proved to be a very effective method for driving medical progress in the twentieth century, to the extent that the emphasis placed by ancient medicine on social health was almost forgotten. This book is about how chronic life-threatening illnesses affect children's health and how they cope with related challenges which in view of their age seem ill-timed and grossly unfair. The central question of their health in terms of wholeness of being turns out to be a very complex issue considering their experiences in Serious Fun Holiday camps. The medical perspective of their health will be inspected before taking on the more complex issues related to quality of life. The chapter heading taken from René Dubos' book 'Mirage of Health' discloses the medical paradigm of health because a mirage represents what is not there. The medical model of health is negative. It is simply an absence of disease. There have been recent attempts to redirect the medical paradigm towards health promotion and the adoption of a healthy lifestyle, but combating the causes of disease remains the physician's foremost ambition. The power of medicine rests with its ability to tackle pathogenesis and eradicate disease. Leriche described health (Canguilhem, 1991:91) as 'life lived in the silence of the organs', which is an accurate account of biological harmony sustained by the self-correcting process of homeostasis. We are unaware of this equilibrium when we are fit and healthy, but become conscious of our different parts such as a gammy leg[1] when homeostatic processes fail to correct local pathologies. Clinical presentations of a disease are approached by the Faculty of Medicine in an orderly way through eliciting symptoms and signs, interpreting these with the aid of biological samples and images, arriving at a diagnosis and prescribing appropriate therapies. This reactive process of biomedicine combats agencies of disease with aplomb as if a pathogenic assessment is all there is to healing. Wise practitioners are aware that clinical medicine has a wider remit of the whole person in society.

Homeostasis: the self-correcting equilibrium of health

It is necessary to take a closer look at homeostasis because you could say that significant and chronic disruption of personal homeostasis is an essential prerequisite for admission to Paul Newman's holiday camps for seriously ill children. The homeostatic deficit is often obvious in these children, and even those who do not have a visible defect their demeanour may be hesitant and uncertain. Their hospital experiences have been upsetting even though the focus of medical treatments has been on restoration of their homeostatic equilibrium. Medical therapeutics are not neglected in the camp, but attention there shifts to a more celebratory form of health.

The core ideal of homeostasis is a harmonious physiological equilibrium. Key insights into this process were proposed by French physiologists in the nineteenth century. In 1859, Claude Bernard first described the extraordinary stability of the body's internal environment, which he called the milieu intérièur. Walter Cannon further developed the concept in 1929, when he recognised that coordinated physiological reactions maintaining these steady states in the body are complicated and peculiar to living organisms. He designated the underlying mechanisms as the process of homeostasis. Thermostats and various other homeostats maintain health measures within a narrow normal range. The principle of homeostatic equilibrium underpinned biological theory and grounded medical advances in the twentieth century. Homeostasis is at the heart and soul of modern medicine and has been extraordinarily successful in advancing new treatments and research. An eminently successful theory in biology easily generalised to adjacent disciplines such as psychology and ethology, so that equilibrium has been understood as the goal of all animal behaviour (Berntson and Cacioppo, 2007). A healthy equilibrium and balance to life chime with admonitions from the Greco-Roman classical tradition and are clearly highly desirable attributes, but the argument proposed here from experiences in Serious Fun camps makes the paradoxical suggestion that an equilibrium of physiological health is neither necessary nor sufficient for a healthy disposition towards living.

Parson's sick role

The social aspect of health is missing in pathological assessments. The problem of illness for society was addressed by Talcott Parsons (1951). There is a remarkable similarity between the functioning of Parson's 'sick role' and the self-regulating mechanism of homeostasis, the underlying principle of pathogenesis. Physiological measures like blood pressure and body temperature along with our biochemistry and haematology are kept remarkably constant by homeostatic mechanisms unless challenged by overwhelming pathologies. Trauma, infection and cancer are among the common explanations that may disrupt homeostasis and upset the silent equilibrium of our physical body. The 'sick role' likewise aims at restoration of equilibrium in society and if that process is successful, the 'sick role' can be cast aside. The 'sick role' carries no blame and describes a validated excuse from social responsibilities, provided the illness has been diagnosed and treated by a medical practitioner. It is a kind of sanctioned deviance from contributing to a constructive role in society, whilst at the same time encouraging recovery. The matter of being sick carries both rights and obligations to promote the smooth running of society.

The theory has been subject to many criticisms and does not in any way suit children with the kind of chronic severe illnesses that serve as criteria for access to Serious Fun Holiday camps. The 'sick role' was above all a mechanism that regarded health as a dichotomy. The doctor's note had to declare whether the patient was sick or healthy. It was a way of regulating sickness for the benefit of a smoothly run society, but at heart it was an unfair oversimplification of health from a social perspective especially if the individual was non-compliant or the illness was chronic. The functional task of the 'sick role' is no longer taken seriously, but it does retain a marginalising effect, which undoubtedly applies to many of the children attending Serious Fun camps. They have been inadvertently separated from their peers without an exit strategy from their 'sick role'.

The consequences for children of both pathogenesis and the marginalising effect of the 'sick role' are very much in evidence at Serious Fun camps. The children there may have various disabilities, but treatment of medical pathologies is peripheral to the kind of health and healing that happens in places like Barretstown, the Hole in the Wall Gang Camp and the Painted Turtle. Life-threatening conditions such as cancer and leukaemia can be trivialised there for a while and permit a different realignment of health. Paul

Newman's great innovation was to have sophisticated medical facilities available on site around the clock. His masterstroke was to give fun names to the amenities and locate them unobtrusively away from the activities. Problems related to the children's serious illnesses must be expertly catered for in the camp, because only then can their physical health deficits be effectively forgotten. There are other camps that offer trendy opportunities for health and happiness such as alternative and complementary medicine, health education, special diets, holistic medicine, aromatherapy and clinical psychology. Serious Fun camps, by contrast, do not innovate any kind of special treatments, but assiduously follow the medicines prescribed by referring hospitals.

Aaron Antonovsky and the sick role

In the 1950s, Antonovsky was a Sociology graduate student in Yale. It took him over twenty years to untangle his ideas on health and stress from Talcott Parsons, the most influential American Sociologist of the time: 'True to the spirit of the quiescent fifties, Parsonian theory…had no room for conflict, tension or stress' (Antonovsky, 1990). Eventually Antonovsky realised that the pathogenic approach that searched for predicaments related to stress was flawed. The Social Readjustment Rating Scale popular at that time assumed that any kind of stress was harmful (Holmes and Rahe, 1967) and produced long lists of life events associated with health risks. This kind of research became obsessed with statistical methodology to make results more reliable, but the fundamental error was an assumption that stressful life events were inherently deleterious to health. Antonovsky eventually realised that challenging events were an unavoidable part of everyone's daily lives and were not necessarily harmful. The link between stress and health had been reduced to an oversimplified social process based on a functional approach to society.

According to functionalism, society is a system of interconnected parts that work together in harmony to maintain a state of balance and social equilibrium, just like the physiological systems of the human body. The 'sick role' was a response by society to ensure social stability in the face of disrupting acute illnesses. It was the social equivalent of homeostasis. Parsons regarded the sick role as a process of sanctioned deviance from a healthy workforce. A sick person had both rights and obligations: rights of exemption from work that were a legitimate excuse for absence plus associated obligations to seek medical help and cooperate with treatment. Functionalism has similarities to homeostasis as it was founded on the basis that a social system was like the stability of different organ systems in the physical body, as noted by Jeffrey Alexander (1987):

> There are models that describe society as a functioning system like the physiological system of the body or the mechanical system of an internal combustion engine.

Homeostasis and the sick role

Contemporary medical practitioners still rely on the principle of homeostasis because it enables them to interpret various laboratory tests. They can regard deviations from established biochemical norms as a failure of homeostasis indicating pathology. The result of the homeostatic inquiry is a dichotomy – it is either normal or abnormal. The medical paradigm of health is a divisive process. The doctor's note must declare that the worker is either sick or healthy. The patient's story – the history of the present complaint – often points to a location that suggests a deficit in a system, which can be checked by clinical examination and further investigations. It is a mechanical approach that works very well by correcting the defect or eliminating a 'spanner in the works'. The medical paradigm is particular, rather than holistic, as it interrogates each system separately. The homeostatic paradigm of pathogenesis provides a clear distinction between health and illness. It dominates clinical practice and health research in the first world. The idea that life-threatening disorders have a precise aetiology that can be eliminated is attractive to a fearful public. Medical discourse in the media tends to be dominated by dramatic threats from ubiquitous pathologies that are assuaged by magic bullet therapies. The difficulty for children with chronic life-threatening illnesses is that there is no magic bullet and only a blunderbuss approach of prolonged treatments that assigns them to a chronic 'sick role', which separates them from their peers.

Pathology and homeostasis

Pathology and its classifications depend on the principle of homeostasis, so that the existence of pathology can be defined in terms of deviation from the norm when the self-correcting constancy of the milieu intérièur cannot be maintained. Failure of biological homeostasis results in pathology that is expressed as disease. Homeostasis operates a closed feedback system with a dichotomous outcome. If the outcome of a biological measure is beyond the norm, the result feeds back to the relevant homeostat. A high temperature will activate thermostatic cooling mechanisms, and osmostats correct deviations in blood chemistry. These homeostats trigger corrective processes, which may restore the constancy of the milieu intérièur or lead to pathological outcomes if correction fails. The goal of homeostasis is a steady state maintained by corrective feedback loops. Whilst the homeostatic principle of health guided medical practice with extraordinary success in the twentieth century, there was less success when the principle was extended to cover behaviour. People assumed that the same process guided patterns of conduct as steered the homeostatic principle of survival: at a fundamental level, we eat when we are hungry and drink when we are thirsty. The idea contaminated modernity as the principle was broadened to cover all interaction with the external world, so that homeostasis was understood as the primary goal of all living systems. Even Gadamer (1996) who portrayed health as an enigma endorsed equilibrium as the invisible concern of health.

Gadamer on health as a restoration of equilibrium

For Gadamer, health is an enigma, but maybe that is because he assumes that a natural equilibrium is the essence of health when he refers to the physician's art of healing:

> What is supposed to emerge from the exercise of the physician's art is simply health, that is, nature itself…the art can allow itself to disappear once the natural equilibrium of health has returned…the doctor's contribution consummates itself by disappearing as soon as the equilibrium of health is restored.
>
> (Gadamer, 1996:34)

It does seem that Gadamer's apologia for the art of healing is about the restoration of homeostasis:

> Medical intervention must be understood as an attempt to restore an equilibrium that has been disturbed.
>
> (Gadamer, 1996:36)

Gadamer does recognise that the sick individual 'falls out' of things, for sickness is not just a loss of equilibrium but also a social and biographical disruption. This goes some way towards recognising the incomplete nature of medical care, as it needs to be a holistic process as well as a restoration of equilibrium. Sick individuals can fall out of their place in life. His analysis falters here for he states that:

> If the restoration of natural equilibrium is successfully accomplished, the miraculous process of convalescence also returns the healthy back into the general equilibrium of life.
>
> (Gadamer, 1996:42)

It may be true that the doctor's art is a matter of withdrawal and setting a person free, which may be the limit of the physician's role. Gadamer states that human life must be released from protective medical care. That is sensible, but his concept of health is limited by prioritising his focus on the equilibrium of life.

Limits to Gadamer's healthy equilibrium

The limitation of Gadamer's emphasis on 'healthy equilibrium' is apparent in Serious Fun experiences. The children are seriously ill when they come to the camp, and they are still seriously ill when they leave. They are not 'restored to equilibrium' in Gadamer's sense, and yet they are positively 'transformed', more healthful. Two Caras recall a camper's embarrassment and anxiety about her leg amputation. When she came to the camp, she wanted to ensure that her disability was masked by wearing a prosthesis all the time; but her playful participation in activities was transformed by the camp experience:

> It was in the summer and there was a girl, when we had kids from Greece as well over here. I can't remember her name and she had a prosthesis on one of her legs, and the whole day travelling had made it swell a little bit, so it was quite painful for her. So, she was in a wheelchair. I think she wore the prosthesis for the first couple of days or something. She was really uncomfortable wearing a prosthesis and being in a wheelchair…Anyway it turned out nobody really cared, she realized that nobody really cared. She was the one only worrying about it. She was in a wheelchair for the rest of the session. She just didn't give a crap about it, because nobody really paid much attention to it. It was really amazing to see how much the first couple of days she'd say Oh God I need to wear my prosthesis.
>
> Off with the prosthesis. Screw that. I am going to go for comfort here. She realized that no one gave a toss. She'd be in a wheelchair and hop around and it was grand, and then the boyfriend would hoot her around.

There is a hint of obfuscation when Gadamer summarises the process of convalescence as a miraculous return to equilibrium. Antonovsky understood that there was more to life than equilibrium. He noted that disease and stress are so ubiquitous that a risk-free ideal of health was a hopeless ambition. His key insight was that the generation of health was independent of and separate from the causes of disease. The medical paradigm of health is a mirage unless it includes Antonovsky's vision. For Antonovsky, health was not just an absence of disease, but a force for living that he called salutogenesis.

Note

1 The etymology of gammy is said to be derived from the Irish word *cam* meaning crooked. It serves well to indicate a part of our anatomy that has become partially estranged from our body, so that we are aware of its awkwardness and failure of seamless function.

4   Salutogenic experiences
Liberating the butterfly

Antonovsky introduced the concept of salutogenesis in 1979, when he became aware from his research that some female holocaust survivors could still enjoy life to the full. There was no direct link between stress and ill health. Stress has a paradoxical component as it can at times be healthful. The children's physical health was unchanged by camp and yet they were visibly enhanced by the experience. The medical paradigm of health is a condition that seeks stability by excluding pathologies, but salutogenesis is a process that generates healthful resources for full engagement with life. Homeostasis maintains physical health whereas heterostasis sustains salutogenesis. The heterostat of salutogenesis is adaptive and seeks an optimal response to changing circumstances. Antonovsky's idea was that testing challenges gave life a sense of coherence because existence became meaningful when stress could be managed and understood. Salutogenesis may explain the disability paradox of a high quality of life despite adverse health experiences

> The kind of health that men desire most is not necessarily a state in which they experience physical vigour and a sense of wellbeing, not even one giving them a long life. It is, instead, the condition best suited to reach goals that each individual formulates for himself...the pursuit of health and happiness is guided by urges which are social rather than biological; urges which are so peculiar to men as to be meaningless for other living things because they are of no importance for the survival of the individual or of the species.
>
> René Dubos: *Mirage of Health*

René Dubos lays out his beliefs on the kind of health that men desire most in *Envoi*, the last section of *Mirage of Health* (1959). It is an extraordinary statement from a microbiologist at a time when the belief in Western Medicine was at its zenith. He boldly states that man's desire for health and happiness is social rather than biological. It is interesting that Antonovsky credits René Dubos as one of his intellectual inspirations in *Health, Stress and Coping* and especially in *Unravelling the Mystery of Health* (Vinje et al., 2017).

Aaron Antonovsky (1923–1994) was a medical sociologist, who was born in America but spent most of his academic life in Israel (Antonovsky and Sagy, 2017). During World War II, he was drafted by the US army to the Pacific. He first visited Israel in 1948 but returned to the States in the 1950s to complete his doctorate in Sociology at Yale. He finally emigrated to Israel in 1960 and began his research career as a medical sociologist with a special interest in the consequences of stress.

Separating salutogenesis from pathogenesis

Antonovsky introduced the concept of salutogenesis in 1979, when he be-came aware from his research that some female holocaust survivors could still enjoy life to the full. Somehow early life experiences had insulated a minority of survivors from being overwhelmed by the horrors of the holocaust. People can stay reasonably healthy despite dreadful experiences. That was the enigma of health that Antonovsky solved by separating the genesis of health from the genesis of pathology. Perhaps it is easier to begin at the end of this quest for holistic health with a claim that social transformations of children with life-threatening illnesses after Serious Fun camp experiences are compatible with the process of salutogenesis.

Antonovsky did not conceive salutogenesis in a eureka moment, but his concept gradually emerged as a solution to dissatisfaction with the generally accepted relationship between stress and pathogenesis. His initial research focus in Israel was on how different illnesses such as multiple sclerosis, cancer and heart disease caused stress. He came to realise that types of illness were unimportant when compared with an individual's coping resources. Health was a variable primarily influenced by what Antonovsky called general resistance resources. Resources of high socio-economic position resist pathogenesis. There were other important personal resources such as early life experiences that shaped a person's ability to overcome not only common daily hassles, but also major stressful life events such as death in a family, job loss or divorce. Antonovsky like everyone else initially understood stress from ill health as a breakdown in homeostasis. The underlying premise of psychological health was the same as physical health: stress is pathological and upsets our equilibrium. The principle of homeostasis is central to understanding recovery from physical disorders, but falls short on any holistic evaluation of health. Homeostasis was understood as the primary goal of all living systems until some researchers recognised the heterostat, which for Antonovsky became the organising principle of salutogenesis.

Heterostasis: the social paradigm of health

A system is a heterostat if it is organised in a way to maximise a specific internal variable (Korotkov, 1998). Heterostasis is not necessary for survival unlike homeostasis, which is essential for life. It is a way of testing our attributes in challenging circumstances. If homeostasis preserves life, then heterostasis enhances life: the former is hoarding, the latter is spending. They are intimately related and interdependent, but it is the heterostatic impulse that enlivens our humanity. Most living systems infrequently or never achieve their optimal potential. It seems more appropriate to define a heterostatic system as one that seeks a maximal condition without necessarily achieving the Holy Grail. Homeostasis is about preserving the status quo, whereas heterostasis is a desire to explore uncertainty and the excitement of possibility. Heterostasis is not associated with a steady-state condition. In general, the internal variable to be maximised will have an upper limit that changes with environmental conditions. Environments like the weather are never static, so that heterostasis cannot be sustained. Homeostasis is the launching platform for heterostasis. This explains why living systems, in seeking the primary goal of heterostasis, devote time and energy to maintain homeostasis.

Health status after camp

The children's physical health was unchanged by the camp. Any homeostatic flaws such as being partially sighted, having limited mobility or kidney failure were unaffected. Yet friends, family and hospital professionals recognised that the children were different. As young adults, these cancer survivors regarded their short Serious Fun camp holiday as a pivotal life experience that re-orientated them towards being more engaged citizens. A Counselor fondly recalls her time as a camper with memories of overcoming daunting challenges:

> You take away the fact that you were able to climb the ropes course and you overcame your fear of heights. Maybe it's the fact that you led a song in front of a lot of people and you overcame your fear of stage fright; or it could be just the fact that you realised that you are not alone facing whatever illness; or you made a new friend, who understands exactly what you have been through.

The change wrought by the camp seemed quite like a re-orientation of their world view, but perhaps it more accurately accords with a reinvigorated desire to live, with an underlying organising principle of risk-taking heterostasis. It is clearly different from biomedical health and its organising principle of risk-averse homeostasis.

Definitions of health

The word 'health' in most languages has according to Szakolczai (2013) a singular etymological origin related to wholeness or integrity. At a more idealistic level, the World Health Organization defined health as 'a state of complete physical, mental, and social well-being and not merely the absence of disease or infirmity' (WHO, 1948). This definition is unrealistic and has the potential to frustrate well-being as it is unattainable. The medical gaze, already described as a mirage, has a narrower focus and concentrates on eliminating pathological faults in anatomy, physiology and biochemistry. Medical health can be declared if clinical examinations, tests and images do not show any abnormality. A clean bill of health for life insurance is still a negative assessment as it only implies an absence of disease. Physical health is important to insurance companies when assessing risk of survival quantified in terms of homeostatic measures, but that kind of assessment lacks any account of heterostasis and joie de vivre.

Last (1997) had a more comprehensive definition with a claim that health was a state of equilibrium between humans and the physical, biological and social environment, compatible with full functional activity; but equilibrium is only part of the story of health. The 1984 World Health definition of health is nearer the mark as it is neither an unattainable goal nor a state of equilibrium, but a resource for humanity to engage with challenges from everyday life in a meaningful way:

> The extent to which an individual or a group is able to realize aspirations and satisfy needs, and to change or cope with the environment. Health is a resource for everyday life, not the objective of living; it is a positive concept, emphasizing social and personal resources as well as physical capabilities.
>
> (WHO, 1984)

The Ottawa charter for health promotion moves beyond health as a resource to salutogenesis – the generation of health through understanding human desire not only to survive but more humanely to live, love, learn, work and play (WHO, 1986):

> Health is created and lived by people within the settings of their everyday life; where they learn, work, play and love. Health is created by caring for oneself and others, by being able to take decisions and have control over one's life circumstances, and by ensuring that the society one lives in creates conditions that allow the attainment of health by all its members.

Health is not the objective of living but a resource for everyday life that assists individuals or groups satisfy their needs (homeostasis) and realise their aspirations (heterostasis).

The health outcome of salutogenesis seems quite like a new world view. Life has a purpose. The salutogenic process induces a belief that personal and social resources will be available to overcome challenging circumstances. The process contrasts with the accepted understanding of biomedical health and its organising principle of homeostasis. The principles of homeostasis and heterostasis are tightly intertwined in the generation of health, but they need to be unpicked separately to clarify their overlapping roles in the enigma of health.

Etymology of salutogenesis

The etymology of salutogenesis means the origin of health. The term *salud* contains an element of celebrating life similar to *sláinte*, the traditional Irish toast for good health. Saluto also contains an element of respectful recognition to a greater power as in salute. It is a celebration of life, whilst recognising the need for good luck as uncertainty is an inevitable consequence to being alive. Ashes to ashes and dust to dust from the *Book of Common Prayer* intones a concise summary of the second law of thermodynamics, sometimes referred to as entropic doom. We have in our lifespan a temporary power to resist entropic doom and side with cosmos over chaos. Salutogenesis in keeping with its etymology is a way of celebrating a meaningful life balanced by recognition of our limited ability to reduce uncertainty. Salutogenic health is more a process of being able to harness personal and social resources relevant to prevailing conditions and thereby engage in challenging social activities that are intensely satisfying and meaningful.

Sense of coherence: the key concept of salutogenesis

Salutogenic health ranges as a continuum from ease to dis-ease. It is a kind of health barometer that reflects an individual's sense of coherence that enables utilisation of available resources. It is a holistic appraisal. In contrast, pathogenic investigations are divisive measures that can only arbitrate in the presence or absence of disease. Antonovsky's initial explanation for a position on the continuum of health was 'availability of resources that could cope with health challenges', but further analysis suggested that there was a single variable that empowered an individual towards the healthy end of the continuum. Antonovsky called this variable the sense of coherence. The salutogenic process directs how our life experiences help shape our sense of coherence to utilise available resources (Antonovsky, 1979).

Antonovsky's concept of salutogenesis has a much wider interpretation of health than that measured by medical tests. His idea was that the origin of health lay with an individual's coherent utilisation of all available resources to generate a meaningful existence. A coherent sense of self could galvanise the optimal use of available resources to overcome stressful situations. Despite repeated challenges, the world still makes sense – it can be understood. It is manageable in a way that invites participation and contributes to a meaningful existence. Antonovsky eventually placed meaningfulness as the most important component of a sense of coherence above understanding and managing the world. A high sense of coherence, the key concept of salutogenesis, enables confident engagement with life, whilst respecting limits to our capacity for creating harmony. The latter is confined by our position in the world – our horizon of expectations. Salutogenesis in keeping with its etymology is a way of celebrating a meaningful life balanced by recognition of our limited ability to reduce uncertainty. It is a holistic way of being in the world that perceives health as a continuous variable fluctuating between ease and dis-ease. There is a modicum of health present even when one is at death's door. Health is then a resource and not a condition. Sick children get this insight by being in a large group with the same illness in Serious Fun camps. They see children who are worse off than themselves and yet participating fully in the activities as noted by a camp graduate:

> You see people worse off and more sick and you say to yourself, if these children are able to do those things what is stopping me.

Before they come to camp they were constrained by a mentality of being unwell which prevented them from participating in the game of life.

The Yale Study Center has collaborated with the Serious Fun Associ-ation for a number of years. They have collected findings on a range of camper attributes and outcomes by requesting parents and caregivers from several Serious Fun camps to complete questionnaires. Their most recent report (Tominey et al., 2015) suggests that the camp releases children from reminders of their illness and builds their capacity for resilience. They used a concept of resilience as an ability to 'bend but not break' (Mastens and Gewirtz, 2006). There are many similarities between resilience and salu-togenesis. Both resilience and a sense of coherence are assets that come un-der the salutogenic umbrella, which serves as a framework that covers many concepts explaining health and a good life (Eriksson and Lindström, 2011). The emphasis in resilience is on homeostatic recovery, whereas salutogen-esis assumes that human nature is predominantly heterostatic. Life is more than survival as indicated by Eriksson and Lindström in the title of their article on the links between salutogenesis and resilience. The Yale Study Center report effectively acknowledges this distinction as it emphasises the heterostatic benefits of social support and relationship skills that accrue from Serious Fun experiences. The heterostatic element of salutogenesis may capture the totality of Serious Fun experiences, whereas a psychologi-cal mentality of resilience, the ability to bounce back, is a variable founded on physiological aspects of coping and psychological aspects of stress (Tusaie and Dyer, 2004). Heterostasis and homeostasis are inextricably linked, but, in general, it can be said that the process of homeostasis is about survival, whereas heterostatic opportunities are linked to quality of life. Theories of salutogenesis and resilience are an arid landscape compared with the lived experience of camp alumni:

> You would never really be able to explain what Barretstown has done. No one could explain what Barretstown did. It was a dream come true. The different people made it as well. I'm crying nearly. Barretstown was just dreams basically. It just comes back to you again and again. You can sit here talking for ten days; you see everyone has different types of expe-riences. If you put them all together there is still something you can't say.

> It's dreams. It's magical. Dreams and hopes, the best experience of your life, it will be the best fun of your life. You can't say it is this or it is that, you have to go and experience it. It would be just beyond anything. You just can't compare it to anything.

When camp alumni were asked to envisage their life without the Barretstown experience, their answer was clear cut:

> You couldn't imagine it it's like somebody trying to imagine being dead. Life would be very different.

There was recognition of children in camp who were worse off than themselves:

> When you come here you see other kids a lot worse off than you and they are able to do those activities. If these children are able to do those things what is stopping me?

Before they come to camp, they were constrained by a mentality of being unwell, which prevented them from participating in the game of life. Then they see in camp the paradox of disability, as sick children like themselves can visibly enjoy and fully participate in the activities.

The disability paradox and quality of life

The disability paradox (Albrecht and Devlieger, 1999) of a high quality of life despite adverse health experiences has frustrated quality-of-life scholars. Albrecht and Devlieger argue for a balance theory of equilibrium between the mind, body and spirit, and claim that a poor quality of life reflects an absence of such a balance. They note the lack of consensus in quality-of-life studies. They suggest that quality of life refers to a holistic notion of well-being and is a broader notion than health-related quality of life. It embraces social, psychological and spiritual well-being. They propose a balanced equilibrium between individuals and their environment as the source of health and quality of life. They draw a parallel between their work and Antonovsky's concept of salutogenesis. They regard salutogenesis as a coherent *weltanschauung* gained by mastery of available resources. Antonovsky's sense of coherence derives from his notions of comprehensibility, manageability and meaningfulness and is, according to Albrecht and Devlieger, equivalent to their concepts of mind, body and spirit. They do not consider Antonovsky's suggestion that homeostasis is the organising principle of pathogenesis, whereas heterostasis is the defining principle of salutogenesis. Their emphasis on equilibrium is hard to reconcile with Antonovsky's reliance on heterostasis. Antonovsky's key contribution was to separate the business of homeostasis (medical care) from heterostasis (meaningful engagement with life). Albrecht and Devlieger remain tied to equilibrium and homeostasis as guiding first principles of health and well-being. Quality of life in this paradigm remains entangled with an assumption that correction of pathogenic upsets should be reflected in quality-of-life measures. They need to consider the heterostatic impulse and its relationship with homeostasis.

Heterostatic–homeostatic relation

The heterostatic–homeostatic relation is a difficult dynamic to chart. The ideal of homeostasis must be Leriche's description of health as the silence of the organs (Canguilhem, 1991). Silent function of the organs means that heterostatic engagement with life will not be thwarted by physical ailments. The homeostatic ideal cannot be sustained, as inevitably there will be pathogenic deficits that require a therapeutic response. The caul of childhood serious illnesses such as cancer can never be fully shed by survivors, as latent possibilities of relapse, second neoplasia and long-term side effects of treatment remain possible (Bhakta et al., 2017). They may in practice return to full homeostatic physiological health, but recovery of well-being is another matter. The consequences of long-term interferences with homeostatic health can be demoted to the point of irrelevance by the camp experience as remarked by an alumnus of the Painted Turtle with chronic severe illness:

> I can tell that I am definitely more confident with myself in general especially with my disease. I am just much more open about it because I realise that there are so many people going through what I am, and I have no reason to be ashamed of it because I am who I am. It's a huge part of me and I have come to love that part of me, as weird as that sounds. It's part of who I am and I can't deny and I can't change it, so you have to embrace it. I think I have – just because I have been here. I see how many people love me for that part of me and how many amazing memories I have and friendships I have made because of that disease. So slowly over time it's been this, I can't even explain it. I am so much more confident with myself. I am happy with who I am and accepting those things that have happened to me. I can't find the words to explain it. It's a slow process over time, but looking back I can definitely feel the change.

Heterostasis has the power to reach beyond homeostatic upsets to a point of sustaining quality of living even in the face of the most extreme disability such as locked-in syndrome (Bruno et al., 2011). This devastating condition has been described beautifully by Jean Bauby (2008) in his autopathography *The Diving Bell and the Butterfly*. His body has been almost completely disabled as if trapped in a diving bell. Despite his total paralysis, he retains a heterostatic urge to communicate his desires – the butterfly within.

The diving bell and the butterfly within

The facts of locked-in syndrome are chilling confirmation of almost total homeostatic failure. In Bauby's case, there is still a fluttering determination to live and be creative. How can this defiance of almost complete disability be explained? Why does his attitude seem illogical? The answer may be found in the twentieth-century error of attributing all health issues on to the single principle of homeostasis. A principle of self-correcting homeostasis serves the medical paradigm of health care very well, but does not suit an understanding of healthful engagement with the social world. To avoid this kind of confusion, Antonovsky suggested that we use disease care instead of health care (Pelikan, 2017), when we refer to the realm of biomedicine.

The fluttering butterfly in Jean Bauby's autopathography can be taken as a metaphor for venturesome living despite complete incapacity of voluntary movement and expression. His debilitating physical ill health was effectively a paralytic imprisonment like living in a diving bell. The book is an unsettling account of difficulties faced after sudden onset of locked-in syndrome. Locked-in syndrome is usually caused by a sudden stroke in the brain stem (Bruno et al., 2011). The brain area affected is small but the effects are profound. Patients retain consciousness despite total body paralysis and inability to speak, though vertical eye movement and blinking are retained and may facilitate communication. The finding that some locked-in syndrome survivors may not want to die counters a popular belief that such patients would be better off dead (Doble et al., 2003). We tend to equate such profound disability with a hopeless prognosis, but a minority can be managed at home with an enhanced desire to live (Smith and Delargy, 2005). In a darker vein, Bauby describes vexed issues he had to face surrounding his quality of life summarised by the paradox in the title of his autopathography. Bauby communicates with his speech therapist through eye movements. He records his memories, longings and final acceptance of his condition (Kearney, 2006):

> In Bauby's case, his illness trajectory terminated with completion of his story. His eloquence is noble in the face of almost complete disability. His resolution inspirational and a statement of great dignity in the face of adversity. The narrative has the power and simplicity of a haiku. Shiki was one of the great practitioners of haiku, those Japanese inspirations of seventeen syllables. He provides a suitable verse:
>
> > Yellow butterfly...
> > Fluttering
> > Fluttering on
> > Over the ocean.

Camp butterfly

The social excitement of Serious Fun camps, akin to a blend of Durkheim's concept of collective effervescence (Durkheim, 1995) and Victor Turner's idea of communitas (Turner, 1969), could be a spontaneous reaction by campers to joyful recognition of belonging to a fellowship, even if it is in the kingdom of the sick (Sontag, 1991). These intense social interactions generate a fluttering sensation of internal nervous excitement described as butterflies in the Oxford English Dictionary. These conditions eventually produce a sense of calm and belonging in the world – a post effervescent harmonic order – a sense of coherence. It is a holistic process as the campers feel healthful despite their childhood experiences of hospitals and life-threatening illnesses.

Bauby's butterfly informs a yearning desire for new possibilities. It is a metaphor for Eros – not a Freudian Eros – but a fluttering desire for a resourceful sense of coherence. Antonovsky's concept of salutogenesis had a much broader interpretation of health than that measured by medical tests. His idea was that origin of health was related to an individual's sense of coherence, which optimised use of available resources. Antonovsky's terminology for the components of coherence was meaningfulness, comprehensibility and manageability – akin to Plato's faculties of mind: feeling, thinking and doing. Through social development, we feel our way into a meaningful world. Speech and language enable thinking and cognitive development. Mobility and manipulation describe our doing and drive our interaction with the world. Plato's trio resonate in reverse with the chronological order of human development as the world unfolds during childhood. Babies are totally dependent at birth, but they slowly become mobile during infancy and develop skilled manipulation. Practical abilities enable engagement with the world through encountering affordances of available resources (Malafouris, 2013). Toddlers absorb their mother tongue and negotiate childhood assisted by speech and language, which are necessary for cognition. Social development of a meaningful world is the most important of the three layers, as it sustains motives to face life's challenges, but does not fully mature until adolescence and early adulthood. Paediatricians assess developmental progress to diagnose biological and social deficits that may benefit from early intervention. Professional assessment of child development seems to anticipate the components of a sense of coherence.

Antonovsky (1987) suggested that a strong sense of coherence is a product of childhood and adolescent experiences. A strong sense of coherence tends to stabilise around the age of thirty with further slight increments into old age. The desiring process of salutogenesis as a coherent wholeness of being in the world accepts health as a continuous variable that ranges from ease of complete health to disintegrating dis-ease. There is a modicum of health present even when one is at death's door. Sick children get this insight by being in a large group with the same illness in Barretstown. They see children who are worse off than themselves and yet participating fully in the activities:

You understand it more with a group of children with same illness. You have a better understanding when you come here. You are protected at home with your parents. You get to play and do all the activities and get to see you can do it. The first time you come down, you would be lost in yourself be afraid of doing things.

Salutogenesis generates a healthy disposition towards the world based on a conviction of being able to use both internal (physical and psychological) and external (social, cultural and economic) resources to achieve a personal sense of coherence. This sensibility allows beliefs that the world can be understood, is manageable and most importantly meaningful even in the face of severe disability and dire circumstances. Salutogenic Eros may trump the encounter with immanent death.

Salutogenesis in Serious Fun camps

Salutogenesis poses the question of health from a perspective that suits this book's interpretation of Serious Fun camp experiences. This might seem strange as it is only the camper's medical condition that permits access to the camp. As a senior advisor to Barretstown said: 'If this is Disney land, the entrance ticket is very severe, and everybody has to hold that same ticket'. Serious Fun camps perhaps more than anywhere else are where these different perspectives of health can be clearly seen. When Antonovsky published 'Health, Stress and Coping' in 1979, he needed a neologism of salutogenesis to reframe the question of health away from pathogenesis. The pathogenic paradigm still dominates medical practice and research whether biological or social, but for Antonovsky that approach could not be correlated with his research findings.

Antonovsky slowly developed his concept. The glaring health disadvantages of poverty raised questions about the stressors of socio-economic status. Stressors cause tension which may be aggravated by lack of psychological, social and cultural resources due to poverty. The issue was resources and not any specific disease such as myocardial infarction. Antonovsky realised that his interest was in the breakdown of health in general and not which specific diseases caused stressful morbidity. There were common factors to all diseases that were countered by a range of resources that distributed health as a social gradient.

Antonovsky's work with concentration camp survivors produced a predictable result in that most survivors were very stressed. Antonovsky's genius was to reframe the question: how did a minority of concentration camp survivors emerge relatively unscathed? The question that Antonovsky sought to answer was the deviant case of those in good health despite hell on earth experiences. The question of how the concentration camp survivors remained healthy could be generalised to: how does anyone stay healthy? That is the question of salutogenesis. Stressors are omnipresent, and denizens of all societies must cope with a range of stressors. Stressors are not necessarily pathogenic because for some the tension of stress can be overcome. A strong sense of coherence supported by appropriate resources may cope with difficult challenges that may become healthy transformative possibilities of renewal rather than a slide down the health gradient.

Quality of life and risk: aversion and addiction

In many ways, children with life-threatening illnesses are immersed in a world of risk aversion. They are wrapped in cotton wool by their families for fear of death or complications. If they are adolescents, they are entering a period when risk is attractive. Risk-taking behaviour is a feature of most societies especially amongst young men. These heterostatic behaviours may be within or outside the law. Bull leaping in Minoan society, modern matadors exhibiting beautiful displays of caping the muleta, climbers that can be seen as mere specks on the sheer rock face of El Capitain in Yosemite, or closer to home so-called joy riders in stolen cars are all examples from different societies of youths deliberately placing themselves in life-threatening situations. They challenge the ultimate reality of their mortality and face the Minotaur. Survival is sweet and makes life meaningful. Risking life is only part of the exuberance of heterostasis as the latter can be achieved in all kinds of challenges from singing and dancing to playing chess. Heterostasis is joie de vivre from participation in activities that are often non-instrumental. Opportunities for heterostasis link to quality of life. The heterostatic effect of camp was recalled by a note in the Harry Potter drawer from a UK camper:

> Barretstown may be the shortest chapter in my life story but it was the most exciting, fun, adventurous, meaningful and certainly the most memorable...I was allowed let the inner childish me out, I was allowed express my immature nature in a positive and constructive way...I am beginning to see things from a whole new perspective which is helpful during day to day life...School is not the same anymore, all I talk about is my amazing time in Barretstown, and of course none of my school friends have any idea what I am barking on about, they think I just went away for a week in Ireland.

Klopf (1972) may have been the first to question the central role of homeostasis in human behaviour. He proposed that the adaptive nature of humans and animals is a heterostatic system. In 1973, Seyle independently proposed heterostasis as a term to cover situations in biology when a feedback system should be reset to a new level. The implication for both researchers was the same: biological systems had a maintenance level of activity and a geared response to changing circumstances.

The adaptive nature of most animals is innate and for a specific environment. Heterostasis can be recognised in the animal kingdom in their specific exuberance of bird song, predators hunting, dolphins challenging the bowsprit or raptors diving towards their prey. The meaning is clear – life is good when their experienced environment agrees with genetic expectations of their species. Heterostatic exuberance is largely genetic in the animal kingdom, but mimetic in humanity. The adaptive nature of humanity lacks a genetic expectation. It is open ended and non-specific as it is moulded post-natally, so that it can adapt to almost any environment including the afterlife. It is culture that specifies the expectations of *Homo sapiens* and sub-consciously mimed in early childhood. Human desire is a carte blanche in the newborn and is largely dictated by imitation of significant others as will be detailed below in Chapter 6 on playful mimesis. Heterostatic theory differs from homeostasis, in that the system seeks a maximal condition as its primary goal – it is a positive feedback loop. A friend of mine used to say, 'it tastes like more'. Addictive behaviour has an element of unbridled heterostasis. The difficulty for humanity is to steer a course between risk aversion and risk addiction.

Klopf's theory of heterostasis does not displace homeostasis at the level of survival, but man does not live by bread alone. Homeostasis still operates in living systems, but it is not the primary goal in humans and remains subordinate to heterostasis. The default state of man's physiology is homeostatic and risk averse, whereas the default state of his value orientation is heterostatic. The condition of heterostasis for any organism is a rare achievement, as it implies that a specific internal variable such as health has achieved its optimal potential. Heterostasis is not necessary for survival unlike homeostasis, which is essential for life. The heterostatic effect of the camp was recalled by a Barretstown graduate:

> I used say to my Ma before I came down here that I'd be better off dead! Mother asked why are you saying things like that? Because you would have no life. Hospitals were my life – you are not allowed to do anything. But then I came down here and when I went home I went crazy.

Heterostasis is joie de vivre from participation in activities that are usually just for pleasure and not task orientated.

Salutogenesis and pathogenesis

Salutogenesis and pathogenesis are separate processes and not unique alternatives for a correct approach to health. They exist in relation to each other, and either can dominate. They can be understood by recognising that homeostasis underpins the status quo, but that is insufficient for flourishing. Flourishing and salutogenesis require a heterostatic disposition. The pathogenic paradigm demands attention to correct diagnosis of flaws, whereas salutogenic frames consider holistic assessments of problems. The salutogenic focus is on the person and not on the disease. In salutogenesis, the well springs of health take priority over the causes of disease. The emphasis is on resources rather than risk factors. The magic bullet has its place in tackling causes of disease, but social interventions such as the laying of hands or an arm around the shoulder may on occasion be as important as they express social inclusion that encourages resourceful coping. Inclusion and encouragement are the essence of Serious Fun camps. A Cara recalls how their encouragement was sufficient to mobilise a young teenager, who came to the camp in a wheelchair:

> I'll never forget when I was here in 2001 and the last session, we had a kid from Spain who could speak very little English, who was fourteen and he was in a wheel chair constantly. We heard through the interpreters that the doctors had given him exercises to try out, but that his mother had not been strong enough or confident enough to hold him up while trying out these exercises. But anyway we started doing them and day ten when it came to getting their certs, that kid walked up to the stage and got his cert. And the place was in floods of tears and there was roars. But it was incredible to see that kid how he did not have the confidence himself when he came on day one, that he could walk.

Antonovsky's key insight was that stress is ubiquitous and not something that can be avoided. Life is a risky business. The question then is not to get rid of stress but how to cope with inevitable stressful challenges that must be met as part of being alive. Furthermore, stress is not necessarily pathogenic. It is often salutogenic and can strengthen a resolve that will assist engagement with future challenges. Stress should not always carry a health warning, as the label depends on how a person interprets the challenge.

Pathogenesis and salutogenesis are not mutually exclusive in the domain of health. There are challenges to health, which are exclusively pathogenic such as pneumococcal pneumonia that requires a specific therapeutic response. There are other healthy challenges such as training for a marathon that are exclusively salutogenic, but many challenges require both a pathogenic defensive reaction and a proactive salutogenic innovation. It is a question of the correct dynamic: salutogenesis should dominate unless consciousness is severely hampered by intensive care conditions that suspend salutogenesis due to sedation, anaesthetic or coma. The pathogenic attitude should be subordinate to a salutogenic approach to life in most disorders even when a medical corrective is appropriate. Maintenance of homeostasis does not equate with health. Homeostasis is helpful but insufficient for salutogenesis.

Salutogenesis and flow

Salutogenesis is a product of a strong sense of coherence facilitated by our innate and acquired resources that Antonovsky (1987) calls generalised resistance resources. Serious Fun experiences are an acquired external resource that may strengthen the campers' sense of coherence. A Barretstown graduate recalls this sense given to him by the experience:

> I came away a totally different person. I wasn't allowed to do sports, my doctors advised me not to. After coming here I'm doing all the sports now. When I went home I tried them all, I took the chance it paid off.

Previous researchers have criticised the sense of coherence concept for being both a resource for and a product of challenging events, but it may imply that our sense of coherence has a dynamic relation with experience. Our sense of coherence is like being part of a hermeneutic circle that can self-tune (Vinje and Mittelmark, 2006) through introspection and reflection on events, which can then reverberate in new experiences that further revise our sense of coherence and so on. Lutz (2009) may have clarified the issue by proposing that a sense of coherence and flow (Csikszentmihalyi, 1991) are aspects of the same phenomenon. Both flow and a sense of coherence are matters of focussed attention – a tunnel vision of engagement with the task in hand that blinkers self-awareness. Life repeatedly throws up challenges that can be interpreted as an opportunity or a threat. A strong sense of coherence tilts engagement with the challenge towards an opportunity for flow, whilst experiences of flow in turn strengthen a sense of coherence – a virtuous circle. Flow is a sense of mastery when challenges are overcome despite stretching participants to the limits of their capability. Lutz envisages flow on a vertical axis and time on a horizontal axis as repeated experiences of flow graph a personal sense of coherence. He regards both flow and a sense of coherence as subjective experiences. Flow experiences accumulate to a sense of coherence, so that flow is more like a snapshot of a cinematic sense of coherence, but they are not strictly subjective experiences as they have an image that can be recognised. The mind is a leaky organ (Clark, 1997) seeping its way into the world. A sense of coherence has a social presence that is a visible product as well as being an internal resource for meeting challenges.

Lutz's proposal to integrate flow and a sense of coherence resolves the issue into a reciprocal relationship. A strong sense of coherence enables flow experiences in the future. Difficult challenging events can be experienced as flow, the synchronic grasp of reality; flow events become embodied as an integrated diachronic sense of coherence. Boys may be effectively prevented from gaining an integrated sense of coherence before a visit to Barretstown, as they are not allowed to encounter challenging experiences. They are constrained by the cotton wool of good intentions if they have haemophilia and are forbidden to play football:

> And then coming here, I was shown I could do stuff. It was me being able to play soccer and not worrying about it. Me being able to work with a team. Me being able to talk with other kids about it. To talk to adults that were not scared of it, specifically males. And that's what did it for me

for the first year, and that's what got me health…I was doing some maths from say from zero to fifteen, years fifteen. The time I spent here is less than one per cent. I'd say that about fifty per cent of my best childhood memories are here.

Memories of flow experiences (the process) gel into a sense of coherence (the resource product) that enables further challenging experiences.

Per ardua ad astra: from disability to quality living

The camping experience is about *per ardua ad astra* – through adversity to the stars. The adversity of *per ardua* has happened in hospitals prior to the camp; the meaningful possibility of aiming at the stars is a consequence of the camp. Campers' new attitudes reveal a meaningful orientation towards a venture-some life even without full recovery. This is the disability paradox which confirms that the constancy of the milieu intérièur in homeostasis is separate from and should not be confused with a salutogenic spirit. Homeostasis needs to be maintained to facilitate the primary goal of a spirited encounter with life – the heterostatic disposition. Positive feedback in heterostasis is the spark of life. Canguilhem (1966) anticipated Klopf's concept of heterostasis when he defined a healthy human being as a living organism that is exceeding its needs, whose aspirations are literally insatiable (Szakolczai, 2010). Het-erostatic exuberance in the animal kingdom happens when genetic expecta-tions are in harmony with experiences of the predicted ecological niche. It is a natural response of restricted scope that cannot imagine circumstances beyond those already coded for survival by the imperceptible process of evo-lution. Animals can only thrive in the ecology that determined their genetic selection. In contrast, humanity lives in a web of mimetic desires (Oughour-lian, 2016) that fluctuate like the weather and mould our expectations to pre-vailing circumstances. The question then is who shapes the mimetic desires of seriously ill children? But it is necessary first to take an overview of the camp experience and how it is structured like a rite of passage.

5   Healing rites of passage

Serious Fun Camps for seriously ill children may have long-term beneficial effects on children with life threatening illnesses. The presented evidence suggests that the experience is a contemporary rite of passage. The different rituals of separation, transition and reaggregation can be identified. The separation from family and civil society is remarkably complete. Established norms no longer prevail in the transitional phase of liminality as campers shed the stigma of illness. Collective effervescence and a fellowship of communitas become the mode of interaction. Barretstown added the dimension of Therapeutic Recreation to the American camp experience. The structured sequences of Therapeutic Recreation serve as an aide mémoire for European Masters of Ceremonies (Caras and Counselors) to facilitate cultural transference of the American Camp experience. Serious Fun experiences can be a life enhancing ritual process for healthy social transformations in chronic severe childhood illnesses

> It's no use going back to yesterday, because I was a different person then.
> Lewis Carroll: *Alice in Wonderland*

A 'rite of passage' is a very popular expression, and like a lot of overused phrases, it has tended to lose its rich meaning and context. Arnold van Gennep published *Les Rites de Passage* in 1909, but a translation was not available to the Anglophone world until 1960. He singled out rites of passage as a special type of ritual, which follow a temporal and spatial sequence of separation, transition and re-integration. Separation was from the everyday world of ordinary routines; transition was about social change; re-integration implied restoration of the socially changed back into an ordered society. He referred to the transitional stage as a liminal period. Victor Turner stumbled on van Gennep's book by chance in 1963 (Thomassen, 2014), while he was in academic limbo between Britain and the USA. It proved to be a revelatory reading for Turner. The concept of liminality, which he developed from van Gennep and published in *The Ritual Process* (1969), illuminated his lifework. Prior to reading van Gennep he formulated his own open-ended process that he called social drama to suit his doctorate research (Turner, 1980). Turner's subsequent work foregrounded liminality as the creative milieu of the social world.

Social drama

Turner's field work in Ndembu villages (Turner, 1975) in North West Rhodesia (Zambia) was conducted in the 1950s when functionalism was the order of the day in social science. The premise of functionalism proposed that the social body was akin to the biological body. The ambition was a social science like natural science with clear cut categories and predictable outcomes. Social science of that ilk needed to research how societies maintain stability and survive in the long term just as homeostasis preserves the status quo in biology, as noted in Chapter 3 about the medical model of health. The structure and agency of society, like anatomy and physiology in biology, were fundamental to social science according to functionalism. In the view of Turner's doctorate supervisors (Deflem, 1991), ritual was subservient to social structure and simply a kind of social glue with a patchwork role to repair social instability. The social structure of the Ndembu had to be addressed first before tackling ritual. Turner (1968) duly investigated the social structure which he found was a combination of matrilineal succession and virilocality (women reside in their husbands' villages). This led to unstable marriages and frequent disputes in the Ndembu villages. And yet for the Turners, the zeitgeist of the Ndembu was not their social structure but the beat of ritual drums, which were heard day in day out (Turner, 1985). Ritual had to be more than a mechanism to enhance solidarity. Ritual drumming for special experiences dominated their social world. Turner's break with functionalism came with his move to a processual approach for social drama, but it took him some time to recognise liminality within ritual experiences as the creative milieu of the social world.

Social drama as a process

Victor Turner claimed that the thespian influence of his mother alerted him to the element of drama in the social life of the Ndembu villages. He noted a clear distinction between normal routines of daily life and sudden eruptions of dramatic time. In dramatic time, behaviour switched from an indicative mood of quiet routine to a subjunctive mood of danger, excitement and possibility. Social dramas followed a process initiated by a *breach* in the quiet order of routine social relationships. The breach caused upsets that could range from unfriendly behaviour to episodes of extreme violence. Overt antagonisms might trigger a *crisis*, responded to by the *redressive machinery* of society. The latter reflect interests of those with an investment in the status quo. Priests, lawyers, soothsayers, elders and other officers of the community seek a judicial process to mediate peace. The redressive machinery may include rites of passage. The *outcome* of social drama may be reconciliation, a material indicator of conflict such as a peace wall between the warring contestants or a resumption of hostilities.

Childhood cancer has elements of social drama, but the immediate cause of upset is not breakdown in social relations but disruption in the natural order of a child's health that has the potential to *breach* the social order in a family.

The breach happens as diagnosis of childhood cancer is invariably shocking and unexpected. The ensuing social drama moves a family into *crisis* mode. The experience of childhood cancer becomes a matter for the whole family, as the problem can ricochet around all household members with a risk of sibling neglect, parental unemployment and family disruption (Gaffney et al., 2006). The social response to crises – *the redressive machinery* – comes in terms of formal support from professionals and informal support from extended family and friends. Psycho-social (Patenaude and Kupst, 2005) is a term that embraces most formal supports provided by different experts such as social workers, clinical psychologists, specialist nurses and various therapists. The *outcome* of previous childhood cancer amongst adult survivors can be problematic. They may remain marginalised from their peers despite support from different experts (Larcombe et al., 2002; Stam, 2005) such as social workers, clinical psychologists, specialist nurses and various therapists. The alumni interview many years after their Barretstown experience articulated how they felt separate from the mainstream of their peers before they came to the camp:

> When I found out I had my illness, I felt alone. I thought I was the only person in the world with the sickness, afraid to talk to people. My mum never understood, there was always trouble.

Social exclusion could be self-imposed as a result of their enforced isolation from their peers or lack of understanding by their friends:

> Before I came I found it was hard to make friends. With the illness, you go to talk about it, they think it is a disease or something they don't want to hang around with you.

Social exclusion was only part of the problem as there was also a feeling of incapacity from being overprotected by their carers and families:

> Before you came here you didn't know a place like this existed. You didn't know you could do all these activities. I was afraid to meet a fella and have a family and all. I used to say to my Ma before I came down here I'd be better off dead.

The social dramatics of cancer treatment do not go away. There is a disordering undertow to a child's life with a life-threatening illness regardless of how treatment is going. Nobody thought of ritual as a correcting force that could reorder experience and restore a child to full re-engagement with life.

Ritual performances

Rituals are characterised by a series of repetitive actions that are often deeply emotional and meaningful. The spoor of ritual can be traced back into the animal kingdom, where certain repetitive performances indicate the valid-ity of relationships. The peculiar forms of ritual in the animal kingdom are a source of fascination, but their expression is predictable and stereotyped. Ritual performances express the animal genotype and there is no room for innovation. Bird and animal rituals may communicate ingrained reproduc-tive signals and rank position within a pecking order. There is a recognisable link between the ritual form in the animal kingdom and the highly varie-gated performances of human ritual, but the sheer complexity and variety of ceremonial and religious rituals contradicts the possibility of any simple analogy between animal and human ritual.

The notion of ritual in medical practice in the twenty-first century carries a hint of pathology or a whiff of witchcraft. Pathological ritual behaviour is a feature of obsessive-compulsive disorders in which stereotypical practices such as hand washing become repetitive, useless and destructive to sociability. Personal rituals may become debilitating and if so help can be sought from mental health professionals. Most medical practitioners consider therapeutic rituals as part of ancient history. The positive therapeutic effects of Serious Fun camps like Barretstown have not been recognised as a paradigm for the power of ritual in rites of passage. Ritual hardly seems to be in the lexicon of the psychologists and the paediatricians who have had an academic interest in camp. The realisation that ritual practice was at the heart of the Barrets-town experience was unexpected in modern Ireland. We had been leaving the world of miracles and fairy tales to folklore. Nonetheless, a ritual passage in a modern guise can explain the efficacy of Barretstown. The surprise is its location on our own doorstep and not in far-flung places. This ritual is part of our contemporary life, and yet not an especially modern or a postmodern custom. It has the hallmark of a universal practice.

There are similarities between Turner's processual descriptions of social drama and a rite of passage. The patterns can be integrated when a rite of passage becomes part of the redressive machinery. The onset of social drama results in a behavioural shift from everyday routine towards disarray. Redres-sive machinery such as a rite of passage reverses the process and moves social life back towards harmony:

> Social life, then, even its apparently quietest moments, is characteristically 'pregnant' with social dramas. It is as though each of us has a 'peace' face and a 'war' face, so that we are programmed for cooperation, but prepared for conflict. The primordial and perennial agonist mode is social drama.
>
> (Turner, 1982:11)

Both social dramas and rites of passage are in the subjunctive mood – the realm of uncertainty and possibility. Social dramas happen out of the blue; they are unpredictable disordering events. In contrast, rituals are deliberate and organised social responses to recent or historical disturbances. Ritual and drama mediate the order–disorder dynamic of society. Rituals can serve as

cautionary reminders of or a solution to the threat of disorder from social crises; rites of passage are social responses that organise some predictability onto
life's crises. The outcome is predetermined in most of the passages because
there is no holding back the underlying natural maturation. During puberty,
boys will become men anyway, but the timing of communal recognition
can be regulated to suit social harmony. In contrast, the outcome of serious
illnesses is uncertain as the direction of individual outcomes may be towards
cure, chronic disorder or death. Illness upsets both natural and social order.
Statistics can provide a probable population response to therapeutic interventions for natural disorders. Significant mean differences between population
outcomes of diverse treatments will dictate a choice of interventions for pop-
ulations, but uncertainty prevails at individual level, as personal recovery may
be anywhere on the Bell curve. The redressive machinery of rituals can placate the problem of uncertainty in the social domain – even when the concern
is mainly to do with recovery from natural disorders. Serious Fun camps are a
kind of redressive machinery that use a rite of passage structure to address the
social disorder associated with potentially fatal childhood conditions.

Ritual as an antidote to suffering

Rappaport (1999) places ritual at the heart of humanity, whilst noting its
biological heritage. Troubled humanity responds in ritual form. Ritual expressions alleviate suffering ranging from repetitive cleaning in obsessive
compulsive disorder to rituals of communal grief that unite a people in settings like memorials of the Great War at the cenotaph, the lowering of flags,
the laying of wreaths and final salutes to honour the fallen. When the Queen
of England came to Ireland in 2011, she was the first British monarch to visit
the Republic for 100 years. There was a coolness to British–Irish relationships
in the intervening century. Hundreds were killed in the Easter uprising of
1916 against the British government. It was easily quashed, whilst at the same
time tens of thousands of Irishmen died in World War I fighting with the
British army. The execution of the 1916 leaders transformed nationalist opinion towards independence and bitter recrimination against Britain. When
the Queen visited the Garden of Remembrance in Dublin, she bowed her
head before the monument to 1916 rebels and laid a wreath in their memory.
Her ritual gesture marked peace between neighbours better than any words
and transformed relationships between Britain and Ireland. Ritual is a potent
process about social formation – to conform, reform and transform tradition.
The fascination of Nuremburg rallies should alert all participants of ritual's
potential for evil as well as good: rituals can deform and malform as well.

Contemporary rituals

Rituals self-assemble when there is a deep social need and, if successful, are
sustained by practice. Self-assembly certainly applies to Serious Fun camps,

even though most of their design, organisation and know-how are inspired by American camp experiences. American camp experiences are taken for granted in the USA, but their unique customs were unfamiliar to Europeans. Their strange holiday camp practices of excluding the real world, their lack of apparent hierarchy, the agenda-free friendliness, the cheerful kindness, the structured achievements and the communal endorsements of success make camp a heavenly place for seriously ill children, but to uninitiated observers seemed an odd affair provoking deep puzzlement. That may be the reason why the camp's rite of passage structure was more easily discerned outside of America, where camp experiences were not taken for granted.

Ritual is a cultural system of standardised behaviours that manipulate human emotion towards a purpose. According to Handelman (1998), rituals are constituted by practice and without practice there are no rituals. Outdated rituals no longer have the power to evoke. Rituals can be judged as social processes that mobilise cultural forms of being such as faith, hope, charity, courage, guile, honesty, grief, endurance and sacrifice in response to communal wants and needs. Ritual performances display these communal forms as an exaggerated agency of harmonic movement and repetitive drills that are often deeply emotional and meaningful. When the monarch declares 'I dub thee knight', it is not simply a promotion, but deeply meaningful as well, for a knighthood carries a social obligation of chivalry. If there is no chivalry, it may mean that the ritual has become outdated.

Serious Fun camps as rites of passage

Turner (1969) grouped rituals into seasonal, contingent and divinatory categories. Rituals may be seasonal, hallowing a culturally defined moment of change in weather, as in a harvest festival. They may be contingent, held in response to great life transitions such as birth, marriage and death: life crisis ceremonies. Contingent rituals may also be rituals of affliction, performed to placate supernatural forces believed to have afflicted villagers with illness. Divinatory rituals are ceremonies performed to ensure health and fertility in human beings, animals and crops. The suggestion here is that Serious Fun Holiday camps are contingent rituals of affliction that are structured like a rite of passage. The tripartite rite of passage experience with its sequence of rites of separation, transition and re-integration can be recognised in Serious Fun camps.

My initial experiences of Serious Fun camps were a mix of strangeness and familiarity. I was familiar with serious life-threatening illnesses like cancer and leukaemia that afflicted the campers, but the strange isolation of the Barretstown camp experience felt like trespassing into the unknowns. The camp sessions coincided with my introduction to an Anthropological strain of Sociology. I had no expectation of a close alignment between theory and practice such as that found in Medicine. The finding of a close association between rite of passage theory and camp experiences was mesmerising. It drew

me into elusive areas of medical practice like quality of life that seem imper-
meable to biomedical science. The American camp experience for seriously
ill children became an elegant demonstration of a rite of passage. That initial
diagnosis produced a eureka moment of surprise, and my initial satisfaction
of agreement between camp routines and theory from Anthropology has kept
me embroiled in the deeper mysteries of camp culture for over a decade. It
is still hard to get to grips with how the USA, the greatest exponent of modernity, has developed and harboured ritual secrets for social transformations
from a bygone age. Serious Fun camps rediscovered ritual healing processes
by serendipity. The camps intuitively found a process which transformed the
lives of seriously ill children as if by 'magic', without realising that they had
reinvented a contingent ritual of affliction structured in the form of a rite of
passage.

The Barretstown experience as healing rites of passage

The focus of this chapter tries to understand and explain Serious Fun experiences. Interviews with administration staff in Europe and the USA suggest
that the experience has many features of a ritual that in other cultures mark
a social process of change (Mandela, 1994).[1] The Barretstown experience can
be interpreted as stages in a rite of passage – separation, transition and re-
aggregation, and the middle stage can be further elaborated into experiences
of liminality and communitas. A rite of passage with its tripartite structure
marks a recognisable cultural change in the passengers such as that happens
in the great transitions of birth, adulthood and death. The different stages can
be interpreted as defining the Serious Fun experience.

The rite of separation

There is strong evidence of separation from the everyday world. Camp locations are all off the beaten track in rural settings and the children do not have
access to the media. All the trappings of modern communication are aban-
doned in favour of close communication with their peers and Counselors or
Caras. The first phase in a rite of passage signifies detachment of the individual from an earlier fixed point in the social structure – the rite of separation.
Serious Fun experiences are exceptional as children with a life-threatening
illness are exiled from home and hospital in a play camp for five to ten days.
Separation of sick children from their home and hospital care for a short
holiday camp experience seems a shocking proposition. The separation from
their everyday routine is remarkably complete. Seriously ill children detach
from previously fixed points in their social structure of family life and all the
social apparatus of care within which the child has been enmeshed for the
duration of treatment. All the trappings of modern communication are aban-
doned in favour of close communication with their peers and Caras. During
that time, they do not have access to their families or friends (no mobile

phones, no texting) and there is no communication with the outside world (no TV, Internet, radio or newspapers). Most children have already separated from their parents and families by the time they reach the castle. The staff in Barretstown only see the endpoint of separation. Many have travelled long distances from as far away as Russia. They are collected at the airport by special buses. They arrive in the 500 acre grounds with a great deal of noise and horn blowing. In Barretstown, they are met at the castle door by great cheers from the assembled staff. They tumble from the buses dazed, tired and bemused. They lose contact with the outside world as described by staff members:

> They arrive rather frightened and shy and certainly very tired. The first day is the shell shock day. The second day is the confusion. What is going on here? And the home sickness comes in on the second day.

The Painted Turtle in California is less intimidating than a castle but the sense of a special space is the same as noted by a counselor:

> It's a wow factor for the kids when they are first arriving: the flags as they walk by, even the archway with the Painted Turtle written on it. You can tell when you are driving through it, it's a different space, you can get goose bumps. I always get goose bumps when I drive up back on the camp. You can tell that it is another special space.

The sense of separation affects not only the children, but also the counselors of the Painted Turtle as well:

> I think whoever decided it should be technology free, no cell phones, no computers, no TV. I hadn't watched the news in years and last inter-cession we were watching the news and it's so depressing I said I need to shut this off. It's awful. It's so depressing. So we have that environment.

The children are deliberately protected in their own little oasis and need to be safely separated from the real world. Senior staff in Barretstown have translated their insights into rules, so that the children are kept separate from visitors to the castle who are not allowed to be spectators of the children's activities:

> I think the freedom they feel in a safe environment not only physically and psychologically but also emotionally, creates the kind of environment where a child feels freer to try things and do things. I think that's one of the most important aspects of this programme that the environment is safe. We will not tour the kids doing activities, simply because the environment here is like a microcosm. The children very quickly in a day or two get used to their staff team, they know the faces they see

around every day; they don't expect to see any strangers and to maintain that level of comfort for the kids is important. We avoid at all times having people walking through, be it on business or whatever, just because you know the children get into an environment where they feel very relaxed and very comfortable.

(Senior Staff Member Barretstown)

The children move away from the encumbrance of illness. They step into the unknown. Doctors, teachers and parents no longer tell them what they can and cannot do. The separation from their previous life is virtually complete. The thoroughness of the separation distinguishes Serious Fun camps from most other kinds of children's camps such as the Boy Scouts (Baden-Powell, 2007), obesity camps (Gately et al., 2005) and even Hitler Youth (Dearn, 2006). These other kinds of camp teach skills or preach ideologies that have practical connections with the real world. Medical specialty camps provide illness-specific education with the intention of promoting health outcomes (Carlson and Cook, 2007). The children's illnesses are an integral part of these camps, whereas Serious Fun camps attempt to sideline the illness for the duration of the camp. As Carlson and Cook (2007) state 'the Hole in the Wall Gang Camps endeavour to take the illness out of the equation'. The counselors of the Painted Turtle supervise camps for several serious childhood illnesses. They are aware of their ability to separate children's camp experience from their illness experiences at home and in hospital, with the single exception of diabetes mellitus:

I suppose the only week that really sticks out for me besides MDA (muscular dystrophy association) would be diabetes week. It's just because diabetes week is really hard compared to other weeks because they have to do checks every so often. It does not feel like normal camp.

(Painted Turtle counselor)

The reason that the diabetic camp is not like the other camps for seriously ill children is that the separation from 'the real world' is incomplete. The counselors recognised the difficulty as a clash between medical and social responsibilities:

The medical stuff comes into the cabins. That I think is what makes it the hardest. The doctors and the nurses are coming up and you are doing carb counts and you are doing that. I think it's hard because it's a lot harder to keep that focus that it's camp, because you are watching them prick their fingers and putting blood into a machine throughout the day; the different stations and worrying about that; it makes you realise what they are going through. It makes it a little harder to make sure that you are focusing on the camp portion while keeping them healthy.

(Painted Turtle counselor)

The separation from the real world into a liminal space is repeatedly interrupted by medical necessities. Painted Turtle counselors were aware that in most circumstances the campers' medical concerns could be confined to the Well Shell, but this was impossible with diabetes. The children's diagnosis was a pervasive presence in the cabins:

> Even the fact you know for that week it's kind of a thing where for us it's that social aspect – the medicine is always in the well shell. When in that first week we had someone with diabetes, maybe because it was those steroids she was on, she developed it, but to have that stuff in cabin all the time, you know I mean like, it just puts you on a different awareness. I think it just shifts your thought processes and medical comes first.
>
> (Painted Turtle counselor)

The hospital world of illness monitoring intruded on the counselors as they needed to be more concerned about the children's diabetes than their camp experiences. It is interesting that most holiday camps for children with diabetes have an educational bias (McAuliffe-Fogarty et al., 2007), as if the only way to cope with the condition is to master it.

The rite of transition

The stage of transition is associated with an experience of liminality. The concept of liminality introduced by Arnold van Gennep and elaborated by Victor Turner has recently been summarised by Thomassen (2014):

> Liminality refers to moments or periods of transition, during which the normal limits of thought, self-understanding and behaviour are relaxed, opening the way to novelty and imagination, construction and destruction.
>
> (Thomassen, 2014:1)

Camp locations disorientate new arrivals as they are foreign places with suspension of all references to home, hospital and school. Time flies for the campers because of their total involvement with activities and new friendships. The experience of liminality upsets the campers' established relationships with themselves and the world. There is self-forgetfulness in their playful dealing with others as they sense their common hospital experiences. Classical rites of passage (van Gennep, 1960:81–82) begin with a period of humiliation experienced by the whole cohort of initiates that undifferentiates any attributes of distinction. Common humiliation served to bond the group and rapidly create great friendships through sharing difficult experiences. There is of course no violence or humiliation of children in Serious Fun camps. Children coming to the camp have already been through the mill: they have all experienced the trials and tribulations of cancer diagnosis and treatment. The levelling achieved by violent humiliation in traditional rites has already happened through their hospital experiences of various invasive treatments and procedures.

Common hospital experiences set the scene in camp for communitas and collective effervescence:

> They don't mind coming out with loads of jargon because people understand it here. Kids will have a full-blown conversation of about these names of drugs that are about ten million words long. They are all yapping away and it's totally fine to do that over the dinner table. Because everybody understands and that's one of the biggest things for kid. That affirmation and feeling that they belong somewhere.
>
> (Barretstown Staff Member)

Attributes of distinction such as social status, race and gender no longer apply. Communitas in the camp is a style of human interaction that may vary from humour, singing, dance and discourse to drawing and stories, but with the recognition that the interactions derive from invigorating happenings and achievements. Collective effervescence is very obvious in the dining hall, which is the nerve centre of Serious Fun camps. Participation in dancing may be gradual, but by day 3 nearly all campers join in with abandon. Illness no longer seems a burden. The camps are a topsy-turvy world where the coercive powers of modern medicine, disease stigma and familial anxiety are temporarily held at bay as noted by Barretstown staff:

> They can also confide with us things about their illness because at home parents might want to keep it secret or whatever from other neighbours.

Layers of medical history interact with playful participation in challenging activities that reveal surprising new insights, intuitions and self-assurance. This experience of liminality – a heady mix of communitas and collective effervescence produces inspirational moments or periods in the camp when previous structures are recast in an innovative way:

> I think what makes the week so special for us is the magic moments we have. It's nothing to do with the illness at all. It's sometimes you have those moments and those connections with kids and it's nothing to do with why they are here. It's you see them experience something, you experience something with them.
>
> (Counselor, Painted Turtle)

The spontaneity of communitas can seldom be maintained for very long. Human beings in groups will always sediment at different rates as free relationships tend to develop a structure: the experience of communitas is fleeting.

Liminality is an in-between situation of being neither here nor there. Turner (1969) suggests that the liminal phase of ritual is an abandonment of the normal structure of society. Normal society is structured and differentiated; it has a hierarchical system of elites and subalterns in contrast to the egalitarian morality of communitas in a rite of passage. Liminality is a no-man's land with time suspended that is lawless, unpredictable and replete with opportunity and danger. This world of unshackled possibilities needs Masters of Ceremonies as they can indicate the way to a disciplined transformation of social order. An individual perspective of liminality fits with Holloman's (1974) description of 'psychic opening'. Holloman describes psychic opening as 'the simultaneous lowering of major defence mechanisms, accompanied by a high degree of receptivity and suggestibility'. She credits the psychic reconfigurations of her world view as a consequence of peak experiences during a workshop with a rite of passage sequence. This outcome was distinct from common rites of passage aimed at change in social status such as boys becoming men. Holloman suggests that a rite of passage subtype may be concerned with 'transformation of an individual's psychological orientation'. Conversion phenomena to particular dogmas such as religious cults are of this type. The workshop in Esalen, an isolated beauty spot in Southern California, provided a liminal context. The workshop deliberately induced strong emotional responses in participants. The 'psychic opening' resulted in the simultaneous lowering of major defence mechanisms, accompanied by a high degree of receptivity and suggestibility. Her prevailing psychic configuration prior to Esalen was rational and scientific: essentially the standard American competitive lifestyle regulated by rights and obligations. Holloman suggests the switch was towards the weltanschauung of Esalen, which was fundamentally charitable with an emphasis on similarities in the world and an avoidance of precise categories. She claimed that such transformations or conversions can occur over a short period of time and are stable into the future. Twomey (2006) suggested that any framework employed to understand the process of conversion needs an ability to recognise liminal conditions, charismatic Masters of Ceremonies and an analysis of the zeitgeist – the spirit of the times. Serious Fun camps operate in liminal spaces with charismatic Masters of Ceremonies and a zeitgeist of the American camp experience. Holloman recognised the liminal conditions of an isolated beauty spot in Southern California, the presence of Masters of Ceremonies and the zeitgeist of Esalen. Tribal rites of passage were all about a change of status, but as Twomey pointed out were subsequently adapted for religious conversions or in Holloman's case a change in world view.

The 'psychic opening' is a perilous occasion as stable structures and identities are temporarily suspended requiring the presence of special guides called Masters of Ceremonies in the classic descriptions of rites of passage. Counselors and Caras, the Masters of Ceremonies in Serious Fun camps, are likewise special guides. They are the key personnel in the completion of a rite of passage that is more akin to a stigma-free psychic reconfiguration than a change of status. In the absence of inspirational guides, there is a risk of tricksters occupying the leadership space and like the pied pipers leading children astray from homely values.

Rite of re-integration

The Caras are aware that re-integration into normal society is not a simple home coming. Camp experiences need to be integrated with their life at home and at hospital as noted by a senior member of staff:

> The last couple of cottage chats are refocusing them externally – preparing them to leave.
>
> Some of the kids don't know how Barretstown has affected them until they go home. They feel more confident with their friends. They don't feel that they are kind of keeping their friends back.

The stage of re-aggregation and reincorporation into society can only be inferred but reports, letters and emails on file suggest that the effect is significant. Notes from parents are especially convincing:

> She had a fantastic time and met some lovely people. She was brave enough to try canoeing and climbing. No mean task when you have only one leg and poor eyesight. I was particularly pleased that she had joined in with some dancing as she has not attempted this since she had her leg amputated so it was a particular triumph for her.

Counselors in the Painted Turtle reflect on the difference between the days of arrival and departure:

> I think watching the kids blossom that come in so shy and don't want to participate in anything; seeing them really come out of their shell is such an amazing thing. They try the things and they don't want to leave and I would hope that their life is forever changed and their perspective on camp and what they can do in the real world is also changed.
>
> Arrival day it's like the overbearing mother like who is talking, like you are after telling me all this stuff. They get to the well shell and she won't just shut up, and the kid is just sitting there silent with arms crossed. The day they come and pick up their kid it's a completely different turn around. The kid won't shut up. They are just bouncing off the wall; they are just so excited to tell their parents everything. And the parents will tell you 'what have you done to them?', 'this is a different kid than we dropped off'.

Transformations may not be dramatic as illustrated by a counselor who accompanied campers on their journey home. She overheard a young camper announce to his parents on arrival:

One of the kids got off the bus and the first thing he said to his parents was 'I tried peas'.

Hardly magic, but could have been very significant for that family.

Serious Fun experiences can be eureka moments or more likely a slow psychic transformation towards a stigma-free world view. The Barretstown experience is a rite of passage that prepares children for an extraordinary re-integration back into society. It has enabled sick children, in a structured way, to shed their former identities, which have been stigmatised by serious illness. The children shed their handicap of Royal Stigma through collective effervescence in a spirit of communitas with fellow travellers, who have been on the same journey of chronic severe illness. Serious Fun experiences move the campers through a series of challenges overseen by Caras and Counselors. These Masters of Ceremonies ensure that the challenges are safe and successfully overcome. These salutogenic experiences are consolidated through evening cottage chats developing their self-confidence and consolidating a new, transformed identity. It is not the identity of a new status. From a medical perspective, there is no status elevation – the children are in status quo – they are still sick children. Their treatment and prognosis has not changed. The story is different from a perspective of holistic health. Serious Fun rites of passage are a resource that can overcome an inability to participate in and understand life as meaningful. The stress of illness can be overcome as they re-enter their everyday lives enabled by salutogenic experiences that can reconfigure their sense of coherence.

Ritual communication and Therapeutic Recreation

Ritual communicates both self-referential and canonical information (Rappaport, 1999). Self-referential information is what the campers have achieved. A child may climb the high ropes, sit on a canoe, make a pot or simply pat a pony on the nose. Their achievements are beyond the limit of their imagined ability. Successful participation in self-referential activities becomes an index of personal change, which may not become fully apparent until they return home as noted by staff:

> When they are at home and have settled, they begin to realise what they learned. They feel different in their home setting.

The second class of information transmitted by ritual is the canon. Canonical messages are encoded from a 'fixed liturgical order' – a kind of moral code of verities that are sacred and cannot be challenged. The fixed liturgical order of Serious Fun is essentially the American camping lifestyle of communitas relationships, the excitement of collective effervescence and personal achievements. Self-referential messages refer to the here and now of camper's achievements, but canonical messages represent universal and eternal orders of how to behave in the world of camp summarised by the mantra of Therapeutic Recreation: 'challenge', 'success', 'reflection' and 'discovery'. Both classes of information are interwoven in camp rituals, so that the canonical stream of Therapeutic Recreation carries the invariant process of the camp spirit, whilst recognition of successful self-referential activities carries variable personal information which the staff know that they can take home:

> They often leave full of self-confidence and bright eyed and bushy tailed. It's very fascinating to watch it.

The Therapeutic Recreation sequence of 'challenge', 'success', 'reflection' and 'discovery' is effectively a simple translation of American camping spirit. It was introduced to Barretstown, Over the Wall, Bator Torbor and other European camps to facilitate transmission of American camp culture to the rest of the world. Therapeutic Recreation is a recognised discipline in the USA (Peterson and Stumbo, 2000). It was imported to Barretstown by one of the first American counselors who had to summarise the camp lifestyle for the Irish Caras. Explication of how to behave is not needed in the American Serious Fun camps, as it is so much part of the general tradition of camp experience in America, but proved to be an invaluable short hand for introducing camp know-how to new staff in Europe. The term Therapeutic Recreation has also been used non-specifically to evaluate all kinds of camp activities for children with chronic illnesses who seek to improve their health whether by education, health management or psycho-social interventions (Walker and Pearman, 2009).

Kiernan et al. (2004) credits specific positive effects on children's well-being to the Therapeutic Recreation programme in Barretstown. Other workers (Kearns and Collins, 2000) support the suggestion that camping programmes enhance well-being when they are situated in natural surroundings and thereby provide a therapeutic landscape. Barretstown would certainly qualify as an appropriate time-out location from stressful situations. Therapeutic landscapes have been researched by Gesler and Kearns (2002) who try and understand the contribution of place to the healing process. Therapeutic landscapes are usually outside everyday experience as, for instance, in sacred pilgrimages, spas and hospitals. Baer and Gesler (2004) suggest that landscapes should be considered beyond exceptional cases, and part of everyday experience. They argue that therapeutic landscapes can become a psychological space to escape from a situation. Even though the circumstances of Barretstown are compatible with a therapeutic landscape, the process there suggests more an active and deliberate intervention for well-being than a supportive therapeutic milieu in the background. Landscapes are regarded as permanent scenarios associated with well-being. On the other hand, passages are transient structures associated with ritual change. Passages may be part of a therapeutic landscape, but are by definition in a secluded spot away from the panorama. Therapeutic landscapes are more in keeping with an appropriate milieu for long-term human development. Landscapes can be considered as a social milieu extérieur for optimal development of a society, whereas passages are a short-term intervention to effect change in our psycho–social milieu intérieur. Turner's concepts of structure and anti-structure (Turner, 1969) reflect the difference between hierarchy and communitas, or that between landscape and a rite of passage.

Weltanschauung transformation: a reinvigorated world view

In Serious Fun camps children slip through the signifying network of classification which have enveloped them as sick patients – the specialised medical jargon of aetiology, diagnosis and treatment that identifies their illness, the schedule of tests, investigations and medical regimes. In the camp, they are gradually released from this classificatory network of signification, or at least it is downgraded to insignificant for the time being:

> It takes by day two evening, come day three morning, they begin to settle in. Then they just begin to totally become themselves. We focus the cottage chats. The first couple of cottage chats in the evening is towards camp – getting them involved. You just see kids kind of gaining a lot more self-confidence, self-esteem. They say they would never have thought that they would have done this before. The feeling that they are not alone, the feeling that they have somebody else is on the same medicine or hasn't any hair either. They just feel that here it's the normality. It's just that sense of belonging here. The way the children totally open up and share things they have never shared before.
>
> (Senior Staff Barretstown)

All the staff recognise the change in the campers. They can see the children changing:

> You can see the transformation in them.

They all tend to have their own interpretation of 'the magic':

> I think the big thing is self-confidence…Some were very quiet and conservative about talking in some of the cottage chats. But now they are willing to initiate conversation.

Sometimes Dads turn up at the gates as they also want to understand how their children have been turned around:

> They weren't able to socialise and now they are. Talking to one of the dads, he said well I wanted to see what happened to my son. Before he

came he wouldn't go to school, he never played out, he was very withdrawn. When he came back he was so different. He wanted to come and experience what he had experienced. There is something really important going on here.

(Senior Staff Barretstown)

At home, the children are confined to the structured, differentiated and often hierarchical system of medical care and then for a short while are liberated into an unstructured and relatively undifferentiated community that offers them possibilities of change guided by Masters of Ceremonies. The transformation may be best described as a change in the children's *weltanschuung*, a stamping of a new world view that embraces their total belief system. For that to happen, campers need a model or an ideal that can be 'stamped' on their being from an image of an ideal model in the short duration of camp.

Note

1 Nelson Mandela (1994) gave a vivid description in his autobiography 'The Long Walk to Freedom' of how he felt fulfilled by his people's customs of a rite of passage to manhood surrounding the circumcision ceremony. His last few days of boyhood were spent with other initiates. A circumcision expert from Gcalekaland used his assegai to change the cohort from boys to men with a single blow on each boy:

> Without a word he took my foreskin, pulled it forward, in a single motion, brought down his assegai. I felt as if fire was shooting through my veins; the pain was so intense that I buried my chin into my chest. Many seconds seemed to pass before I remembered the cry, and I then recovered and called out, '*Ndiyindoda!*'

In Mandela's story, the transformation to '*Ndiyindoda*'!, ('I am a man!') is a momentous occasion, whereas transformations in Serious Fun camps are more of a cumulative process that continues at home. Mandela's transition closes with communal recognition of his new status:

> I had now taken the essential step in the life of every Xhosa man. Now, I might marry, set up my own home, and plow my own field. I could now be admitted to the councils of the community; my words would be taken seriously.

6   Genesis and mimesis

Caras and Counselors as Masters of Ceremonies have to be radically different from campers. They have left school and ventured into the world. Their many experiences of life fire the campers' imagination. Unlike the children they have exuberant health and energy. In the liminality of camp these young Masters of Ceremonies guide ill children towards unimagined achievements in various activities. They quietly supervise behaviour and lead their reflections. They are a life-long pivotal influence on the children despite the short duration of camp. The campers' memories of their Caras and Counselors resonates with René Girard's mimetic theory of desire, which claims that our desires are borrowed from other people. Mimesis in early child development reprises Merlin Donald's suggestion that mimetic cultures preceded genesis of speech in early hominids. It also suggests how mimetic transformations can happen in Serious Fun camps. Rites of Passage are optimal circumstances for mimetic lifestyle transformations as they can stage transient liminality

> Imitation is often thought of as a low-level, cognitively undemanding, even childish form of behaviour, but recent work across a variety of sciences argues that imitation is a natural ability that grafts our nature to the prevailing culture of language lifestyle and social interaction before the finishing school of rational intelligence.
>
> S. Hurley and N. Chater. *Perspectives on Imitation: From Neuroscience to Social Science*

This chapter is about the role of Counselors and Caras in Serious Fun camps and how in a matter of days they have such a profound impact on the children under their care. A later chapter will look at the alignment of coincidences in 1988 that were necessary to understand how the Hole in the Wall Gang Camp in Connecticut established a life-changing pattern of care for seriously ill children. One of the remarkable aspects of that camp was how they got the ethos right from the word go. They not only got it right but were able to export this very American experience to a different culture six years later.

Counselors and Caras care for sick children while they are in the camp. The titles of Counselors in America and Caras in Ireland disguise their role:

it is what Anthropologists such as van Gennep and Turner call 'Masters of Ceremonies'. The American spelling of counselor in the Merriam-Webster dictionary is absent from the Oxford English Dictionary (OED). Counselor with a single 'l' is closely associated with summer camps in the USA, whilst the OED spelling of counsellor is more connected to marriage and psychological counselling. The OED points to further confusion as their spelling of counsellor is often mistaken for councillor meaning a member of a council. Both the American and British terms convey the notion of advisor, but neither spelling worked well for those responsible for the first European camp as the term seemed too serious and officious. The name chosen instead was 'Cara', the Irish for friend and the designation has been well accepted. Caras have roles as the children's guardians in the cottages, their home for the duration of the camp, and as activity leaders who guide the children in their chosen challenges of the day. If Serious Fun camps are rites of passage, then the Caras and Counselors are undoubtedly Masters of Ceremonies.

Masters of Ceremonies are not 'friends', at least not in the popular sense of the word. Masters of Ceremonies, as understood in Anthropology are first and foremost 'elders', who possess a special knowledge, experience and wisdom. They are special people who have already experienced rituals and presided over several rites of passage. Priests, Shamans, Rabbis and Midwives are all Masters of Ceremonies who occupy positions of structural distance from the neophytes. In some instances, Masters of Ceremonies may be closer in age to the neophytes than in the typical rituals of Shamans, but they will always differ very significantly from them in terms of their knowledge and experience. Former campers may return as Caras and Counselors and most camps have special leaders in training programmes to facilitate that elevation of status. A Master of Ceremonies is a 'friend' to the initiand in the rather specialised sense that they are a powerful agent who is present at a time of need, someone in a position of authority who is friendly towards the best interests of the vulnerable neophyte. The American word counselor retains these connotations of elevation, authority, wisdom and experience, whilst being friendly towards the neophyte's interests. Caras do not necessarily carry the same connotations, but there is the distance of another language. Caras and Counselors as Masters of Ceremonies are radically different from the campers. They have left school and ventured into the world. They have had many experiences of life that are almost beyond the imagination of the campers. In contrast to the children, they have exuberant health and energy that excites the campers. In the cottages and cabins, the only rooms that are off limits for the campers are those occupied by their Caras and Counselors. The campers retain vivid memories of their Caras and Counselors. They are like a Guardian Angel that is someone who is their special friend, but who also has access to the powers that be.

The ratio of Caras and Counselors to campers is at least 1:2, and often closer to 1:1 when other voluntary helpers are included. In the liminality of camp, these young Masters of Ceremonies guide ill children towards unimagined achievements in various activities. They also quietly supervise behaviour and lead their reflections in cottage chats at the end of the day.

Role models

All staff of Serious Fun camps are aware that the experience has a profound effect on children, but the nature of 'the magic' has remained a mystery. Interviews with camp alumni as adults in Barretstown and the Painted Turtle pointed in the same direction. The Caras and the Counselors were a lifelong pivotal influence on the children despite the short duration of the camp. The unanswered question was how role models could achieve a profound effect in such a short time. In Barretstown, Cara volunteers are coached to be proactive role models and mentors for the brief duration of the camp as can be taken from the VALU mnemonic used in training:

> For the duration of camp, volunteers are role model mentors and a reliable sounding board for the children. Mentoring is generally considered to be a process of guided interaction over a long period of time. The mentoring at Barretstown must be concentrated into a period of less than ten days. The volunteer training recommends a language and uses a mnemonic VALU (Validation, Asking, Listening, Understanding) to illustrate how they should care for the children in an exemplary way. Children may easily get frustrated and overwhelmed by imagined demands of the activities. The VALU approach deflects immediate problem solving to an emphasis on individual strengths. It begins with Validation of the child's approach to the activity. Asking starts with exploratory questions of their interests accompanied by attentive listening using non-inquisitorial remarks such as 'tell me more'. The attentive process is crucial as children are ultra-sensitive to the Listening mode of their Cara. Listening should be embodied by engaging at eye level and anchoring. Anchoring is a posture and a demonstration that the listener is not going anywhere: 'I really want to hear what you are saying'. The final part of valu is Understanding as the Caras check back with the camper that their interpretation of the issue is correct. The problem is restated 'Is this right?' Then the Cara can proceed to problem solving.
>
> (Notes taken during Volunteer Training, Barretstown, February 2011)

Caras and Counselors may have the important responsibility of being the sick children's caretakers for the duration of the camp, but for the children they were their *Anam Caras* (Soul Mates) as can be gleaned from their adult memories of their Caras:

> They were always there for you and made us feel special. They make us something and they always had time for each individual. It was never I'll talk to you later…They were like your family and always asked how you

felt. It was like you knew them all your life… They were so easy to talk to. If you had any problems they would understand. They would sit there and listen.

Here is another perspective from a Cara group interview as they spoke amongst themselves about the children during camp:

They note how this kid did really well and went really high on high ropes, or this kid is after doing a masterpiece in arts and crafts; or observing how the children's confidence is boosted through getting that pat on the shoulder and getting them to realise 'yea I really did do something'.

Then there is the reflexivity of cottage chats as Caras and campers reiterate the activities at the end of the day. They remember highlights and what the children liked and did not like. They sit around a fire and if you want to talk you hold the teddy that is being passed around. The Caras noted:

It's up to the children to discover themselves and learn what strengths they have. The Caras understood that the children were making realizations of what they had achieved through little revelations about things going inside their heads about self-esteem. The children realised as a group that other people were having the same experiences as themselves. The children began to have deep chats amongst themselves. They had absolutely massive heart to heart talks as they began to feel open enough to talk to each other.

Camp alumni of the Painted Turtle remembered the relationships they had with their counselors and the impact that made on them. These Painted Turtle campers were now back as counselors:

I would say that because of the relationship I had with my counselors and they were so great and so supportive like that's why I came back and I wanted to be that to someone else. I wanted to make that big difference.

The mentoring process was profound as it influenced their life dreams and ambitions:

The counselors wouldn't treat me as someone with an illness. They would look at me for my characteristics, my personality, my dreams and ambitions. I think it was the way that they treated me and really became interested who I was, yeah, they are the reason that I am here today; because I wanted to continue that tradition and show these kids that they have more to life than the illness that they have.

A fellow camper in the Painted Turtle agrees:

> I want to be the counselor that changed my life. I want to become the new generation of counselors who can impact someone's life for the better.

Behaviour management

Behaviour management was not part of Newman's vision for the Hole in the Wall Gang Camp. His idea was that sick children were just like normal children, but they were unable to play because of their illness and prolonged hospitalisations. These children needed a special camp where they could play, with sophisticated medical facilities available around the clock that ensured their health and safety. Newman wanted the environment to be as non-clinical as possible with unobtrusive medical facilities. That was the case until five years into the programme when the camp had to deal with severe behaviour difficulty in a young man who got angry and upset, and almost made it to highway forty-four. They needed advice. They consulted a child psychologist from Yale University Child Centre. She noted that:

> Cancer does not have any favourites as far as demographics. Most of our kids are not from the inner city. Then in 1993 they began to add Sickle Cell and HIV, which are two diagnoses tied to a less fortunate socio-economic status... These are not children with just medical needs. It may be more helpful to see them as children with special needs, rather than normal children who happen to be sick. We were seeing more and more of a population with children with more than one problem...I got them on board with the behaviour management program that was really focused on intervening as minimally as possible and only addressing issues of safety.

Not everyone was happy:

> Howard Pearson said we don't want any shrinks here at camp. We are not doing therapy, we hesitate to bring in people from the academic community. We had a social worker here and that didn't work out. We had a pastoral counsellor here, they didn't like that.

The child psychologist wanted to know what the non-negotiable rules of camp were. She believed that children cannot play until they feel safe and, together with the camp director, they developed three non-negotiable rules:

1 No physical violence.
2 No emotional harassment – no killer statements.
3 No unsupervised activities.

She claimed that some rules were necessary, but you can still say:

> that you are not doing therapy at Hole in the Wall, but what you are do-
> ing is therapeutic...In the beginning at least Mr Newman and Howard
> Pearson were very adamant that we are not doing research on these kids,
> that we are not therapizing these kids and that we are not going to ask
> campers to fill out questionnaires. This is a free gift.

The three rules formed the basis of behaviour management, which is common
to all camps. In the Painted Turtle, the counselors learn a set of simple ploys
during training that are non-adversarial and maintain a positive approach:

> I think one of the great things about the training is they give you so
> many different ways – like plan ignore, hurdle hugging, redirection. Plan
> ignore is if a kid is doing something and you know they are kind of do-
> ing it just to get your attention. If you ignore it they will stop doing it,
> because they are just doing it to get your attention. Hurdle hopping is
> where a kid says 'I don't want to do anything in woodshop because it's
> too hard to make a bird house.' Maybe if you draw one of the lines on a
> piece of wood they would draw the other and it gets them going. Redi-
> rection is when what you are talking about that is not appropriate 'Oh
> my God look at those kids playing basketball' – just changing the subject.
>
> We don't say no a lot. We don't say don't do this. We phrase it a posi-
> tive way so that they don't really realise that there are rules, and that we
> are telling them to do something.

In general, the campers have a deep respect for the place and they tend to
chide those who get too out of line: 'look that is not cool, you can do that
at home but it's not cool to do that here'. It is a much easier role than being
a parent or a teacher as the focus is on behaviour management for a week
and not about reform. If the techniques are not working, there are support
staff specifically trained, who have professional skills that are occasionally
necessary. The positive approach ensures that campers tend to revere their
counselors, who recognise that they are role models:

> If they are return campers I remember asking a particular camper what's
> your best memory from last summer, and the first response was 'my
> counselor'. And she idolised her counselor.
>
> I think whether one wants to be a role model or not, it's happening.
> We are the ones who are taking them everywhere. We are the ones who
> are facilitating everything. If we're not into it, they are not into it.

Mimesis of role models

The campers' memories of their Caras and Counselors resonate with René
Girard's mimetic theory (Girard, 1996). The mimetic capacity in humanity seems inexhaustible. It has an immense subconscious power to transform

and coordinate beliefs, intentions and desires. Mimesis is the Greek term for imitation and has in recent times found application in both the arts and the sciences. For a long time, imitation was regarded as a playful process confined to childhood and not a matter for serious debate. Since then, mimetic behaviour has been promoted from the kindergarten to the academy as implied by the opening quotation from Hurley and Chater. They suggest that natural abilities of mimetic desire in social situations 'grafts our nature to the prevailing culture'. Mimesis is a two-way street: we subconsciously imitate admired others and in turn inspire others through our lifestyle. The disciplines that have adopted mimesis as a natural ability are many and include Neuroscience, Social Psychology, Anthropology, Child Development and Literary Theory. It has become a key concept in understanding *Homo sapiens*. According to Merlin Donald (2005), there are overlapping levels of imitation ranging from mimicry, through imitation to mimesis. Mimicry, the simplest term is speaking like a parrot – a thoughtless copy, whereas imitation copies the purpose of action as well. Mimesis, the most complex form of reduplication, communicates action with creative representations as happens in pretend play.

The mimetic aperture

Rites of passage are optimal circumstances for mimetic lifestyle transformations as they provide a means of staging transient liminality. Serious Fun camps provide ideal conditions for healing rites of passage. The control of our mimetic aperture may be one of the keys to understanding why some circumstances predispose to powerful social transformations. In some situations, we are open to mimesis and susceptible to subconscious imitation of another's way of being. Then in other places, we close down and are impervious to circumstances. Our mimetic lens is not a constant filter but seems to work like a highly reactive pupil that constricts and dilates in response to local conditions and personal circumstances. It seems to be mainly wide open in early childhood, but becomes much more selective with the wisdom of old age. Youth and ritual make us porous to subconsciously mime lifestyles and world views. The circumstances of Serious Fun camps facilitate the dismantling of hospital conventions and experiences through a sense of camper camaraderie and intense relationships with revered mentors. These circumstances coupled to a wide-open mimetic aperture make campers ready for a change of life course. Mimetic power is neither benign nor malign, but a process that can be used for good or ill. Spariosu (1997) in *The Wreath of Wild Olives* distinguished agenda-free programmes of creative mimesis play from the indoctrination of mimesis imitation, and will be discussed in the section about 'the spirit of the camp embrace' in Chapter 9.

René Girard uncovered the power of mimesis through biblical and literary scholarship, but the subtlety and nuances of mimetic influences at interpersonal level need further study. Mimesis may bridge the divide between arts and science as Girard's findings have been supported by recent research in neurophysiology (Gallese, 2009). Natural scientists have discovered mirror neurons that provide an instantaneous short circuit between perception and action. Mirror neurons can both perceive and re-enact. They may be a synapse-free locus of mimesis in the brain. The full impact of mimesis on social transformations will take multi-disciplinary studies to unravel the subtlety of mimetic power.

Mimesis in evolution: missing links

Merlin Donald (1991) suggested that early hominids communicated in mimetic cultures long before *Homo sapiens* had language. He believes that evolutionary change from chimpanzees, who have at best a very sparse culture, to *Homo sapiens*, with rich and complex cultures, was via extinct missing links who communicated in vibrant mimetic cultures. They did not have speech, but could communicate with one another like mime artists. The camps in Barretstown are often multinational and the lingua franca is not necessarily English. They still communicate very well with one another through mime that is full of humour and creativity. The idea of mime is important because it enables a better understanding of the way we still subconsciously communicate emotions with one another.

Evolutionary innovations in communication do not displace older ways of relating, but instead accumulate in layers. The unfolding dynamic of human development can be imagined by the famous theory of Ernst Haeckel (1834–1919), who suggested that ontogeny recapitulates phylogeny or, in other words, development replays the strata of evolution. The theory fell into disrepute but has re-surfaced and gained credence through human genome research, which has traced our genes back through the animal kingdom, the reptilian world and plant life. Fossils store hints of evolutionary change, but more dynamic insights may be obtained from ontogeny by observations during child development.

Mimesis and child development: ontogenesis

Neuroscience has demonstrated a principle of 'use it or lose it'. The brain of the newborn has myriads of connections that are pruned in response to experiences during infancy. The process is like what happened when a philanthropist endowed a New England campus with several new buildings. They planted grass, but did not lay paths for a few semesters. The ways between buildings were determined by use and the paths were laid. The analogy is crude but the principle holds; we are a hybrid species of our inherited nature and cultural experiences. Experiences shape the connections of our developing brains. The brain in utero develops according to a genetic code facilitated by maternal health. The infant's social world in harmony with the prevailing culture helps shape the enormous development of the brain in early childhood. Postnatal development intertwines the remaining genetic expression of brain development with local inheritance of tradition. Lamarck, who espoused the inheritance of acquired characteristics, meets Darwin's natural inheritance during infancy. Child development traces the interaction between an emerging brain and immersion in a social context. The phylogeny of culture differs from that of biology. The finishing schools of culture that shape our taken-for-granted manners have in the main been lost to prehistory, so there is no precise phylum, but recent cultural pedigrees can be traced through historical records (Elias, 2000) and the artefacts of archaeology (Malafouris, 2013). The newborn baby is an unfinished product and, unlike the rest of the animal kingdom, needs cultural input for complete formation. Infants are pluripotential polymaths that get channelled by the prevailing culture. From an evolutionary perspective, mimetic means of communication in the visible process of human development hints at ancient ways of being in our extinct prelinguistic ancestors. Missing links have become extinct but Merlin Donald (1991) surmises that their intense ways of emotional being and communication are still part of humanity. Emotional mimetic communication can be easily observed in early childhood and in the transient liminality of Serious Fun camps.

Mimesis and paediatrics

Paediatricians are aware that newborn babies have a bundle of special reflexes, which slowly disappear under the influence of higher centres during infancy. Primary walking, the grasp reflex and the Moro reflex amongst others can be elicited soon after birth to impress proud parents. They provide a kind of antenatal physiotherapy as can be seen when these reflexes are weak or absent in utero. Joints become permanently deformed and dislocated in a condition called arthrogryposis multiplex. Despite this knowledge, it was a surprise to Paediatricians as well as Clinical Psychologists when Meltzoff and Moore (1977) published their findings of mimetic reflexes in the newborn. The mimetic faculty is innate and influential from birth. A mimetic reflex is not the same as deliberate mime, but they are related in the way that the neonatal primary walking reflex has a crude relationship with stylish adult gaits. Observations from the nursery rather than the laboratory endorse the importance of mimetic communication during infancy. Reflex dyadic exchanges commence soon after birth, which are soon enhanced by emotional mimesis: s/he smiled! Reciprocal imitation through smiling, laughing and cooing dominates communication during early infancy. Facial expressions, babbling, body language, gestures and pointing are early forms of mimetic communication, which anticipate the development of speech. These expressions reprise Donald's suggestion of symbolic mimetic cultures preceding language acquisition. The subconscious power of mimetic communication shaping child development is evident during infancy. Toddlers remain immersed in a culture of mimetic communication that is a necessary antecedent to the acquisition of speech. It is the same in Serious Fun camps, where communal encouragement and exemplary behaviour by revered counselors impress their charges with possibilities of recovery and re-engagement with life.

Early genesis and later mimesis: learning to walk

The in utero posture of foetal flexion gradually extends during infancy. The baby's core unfolds from head to toe over the first year. The head becomes a periscope as the neck stabilises in early infancy, then the back straightens for independent sitting, and finally, the lower limbs become upright. It takes twelve months to establish an independent stance. At the same time, the hands become fully operational as the forelimbs are liberated from crawling mobility. Genetic programmes equip the newborn with a very crude approximation of final aptitudes. The innate sequence of the stepping reflex in the newborn parodies graceful ambulation in a crude robotic way. It eventually serves as a template for the broad-based steps of toddlers. First steps are just like a drunken sailor whose balance has been compromised by intoxication. The sailor's coordination may recover overnight, but toddlers need a year or two of walking experiences to transform their ambulation from staggering to free running. Personal experiences of the world refine the gait, so that the impulse to mobility may eventually become graceful movements in ballet dancers or effortless sprinting in champion athletes. Even our own mobility is subject to the finishing school of social and cultural environments. There is an American walk, and in Cork we acquire 'a gatch', 'a swagger, a distinctive gait' (Beecher, 1991). The Cork swagger may take some time to perfect, but, in Serious Fun camps, the children's demeanour may be changed in a matter of days. Previously unimagined experiences mime new possibilities and provide the key to unlock the mystery of social transformations in infancy and Serious Fun camps. The whole orchestration of ontogenesis is a delicate and complex matter of wheels within wheels. Mimesis can work its magic in jig time if the mimetic aperture is wide open in an atmosphere of encouragement. Children are often very shy and embarrassed when they come to the camp until their mimetic aperture dilates. A Cara noted such a child, who metaphorically speaking was barely able to swim in the river of life, but was river dancing by the end of the camp:

> I had a girl in one of my cottages last year and day one she was so self-conscious. Like when they were changing into their pyjamas, she would like go into the bathroom and change. She'd like sleep in her clothes rather than let other children see her. And day ten the night before they were leaving, she ran out into the lounge in her underwear – like sign my book, sign my book.

Her behaviour was transformed by the kindness of others. I learned in the Painted Turtle that RAKs were random acts of kindness, and were part of the spirit of camp as an unwritten policy. We are attuned to being impressed (through the mimetic apparatus) by the behaviour of others. Children intuitively interpret the mimes of smiles and frowns immediately – an early form of mind reading – that can later mature into the business of portrait painters.[1] We recognise the mimes of bullies and kindness in a flash. That is what happens in Serious Fun camps when children who have been inadvertently excluded by their illness prior to camp are suddenly faced with an overwhelming lifestyle of kindness, understanding and personal achievements.

Mimetic communication of the prevailing zeitgeist

The entirety of development is a seamless process of ontogenesis, whereby the full capacity of humanity emerges during childhood. The genetic inheritance of evolution must engage with the prevailing social and cultural milieu. Mimetic abilities receive, transmit and create signals as they graft our nature on to the prevailing culture. Mimetic communication connotes impressions and multiple meanings, so that its imprecision and ambiguity encourage humour and metaphor. Local mimetic cultures have a strong emotional grasp on communities, even if it is ill defined and imprecise. Mimetic forms can express deeply held cultural values in all-embracing emotional rituals, most often seen nowadays in sporting stadiums.

Mimetic signs are concrete and therefore confined to the present. They can be symbolic as in a 'shoulder shrug' as well as being indexical and iconic. Symbols are the most abstract form in Peirce's classification of signs. According to Peirce, a sign can be an index, an icon or a symbol (Hoopes, 1991). An index like the finger point is part of what it indicates; an icon resembles the signified, whereas a symbol is an arbitrary association making it meaningless without an interpreter. The emergence of high-speed symbolic language in *Homo sapiens* allowed denotation and precise communication. Language enabled accurate memories of the past and forecasts of the future. *Homo sapiens* was no longer confined to the present. Categorical precision and clockwork time enhance commercial life and military discipline, but Serious Fun camps discard mundane accuracy in favour of fun through communitas in a kind of sacred time. Mimetic communication is the order of the day in the camp through challenging activities and dancing in the dining hall, whilst memories are consolidated through the precision of late night cottage chats. Seriously ill children subconsciously imbibe the spirit of camp.

Mimesis of apprenticeship and appropriation:
Eros of mimetic humanity

Imitation has long been recognised as crucial for children learning speech and manners. It is the age-old way we acquire our mother tongue and local customs. Our thoughts and desires are mirrored into one another. According to Girard, mimesis underpins our cultural apprenticeship whereby we acquire speech, social skills and conventions (Fleming, 2004). This mimesis of apprenticeship is a partially conscious process of socialisation and encultura-tion (Girard, 1996). Learning our mother tongue is a covert process, but can be made overt as the gestation and birth of words can be heard and recorded (Roy, 2009). *Homo sapiens* shares a desire for approval through mimesis of apprenticeship with some social animals. Anyone who has watched sheepdog trials of dogs, which shepherd their flock through gates and hazards in re-sponse to their master's whistle, can see the outcome of an apprenticeship of mimetic desire in another social animal. Girard's great contribution was to recognise a more fundamental operation, whereby subconscious human de-sires (Eros) are acquired by mimesis of appropriation. Apprenticeship is about practical skills, but appropriation of desires is about lifestyle and salutogenesis. The Eros of humans – our open-ended mimetic desire to appropriate our identity and values from others – seems unique to our conspecifics. We do this through social interaction with the modern equivalent of our tribe. Gi-rard sees mimesis as the most fundamental characteristic of human behaviour. His great insight was to recognise mimesis of appropriation in addition to mimesis of apprenticeship. This recognition identified desire as the mimetic force. Eros is not an internal Freudian appetite, but an external mimetic han-kering conducted from afar – a mimesis of desiring appropriation ranging from rivalry to reverence. Mimesis nourishes dynamic interactions between a culture and its inhabitants. Mimetic desire can be grafted on to appetites, but it can also emerge completely independent of biological needs. Humanity is a dedicated follower of fashion that is fickle and irrational. Potent human desires tend to emerge when basic appetites of existence are satisfied:

> Once his basic needs are satisfied (indeed sometimes even before), man is subject to intense desires, though he may not know precisely for what. The reason is that he desires being, something he himself lacks and which some other person seems to possess. The subject thus looks to that other person to inform him what he should desire in order to acquire that being.
>
> (Girard, 1977:146)

The desires of sick children, unlike their healthy peers, are likely to be cur-tailed by the demands of their illness. They see in their Caras and Counselors an exemplary fullness of being that is beyond the bounds of their imagined future. Graduates of the Painted Turtle have fond memories of their counse-lors and recall that fullness of being:

> I just remember being the oldest campers; I became friends with my counselors. They became friends to me and we would just communicate like one on one, equal levels, just talking about our lives; but also they were such great mentors. Just hearing about their plans, going to med-ical school, going on mission trips or just travelling the world, it was so inspiring to me, even at fifteen and sixteen I realised that the world was totally open to me; I could do whatever I wanted to do. They put so

many new goals and inspirations into my head. It was just amazing to get to know them and build relationships with them, a lot that I still have to this day with a lot of the counselors.

Eros can be driven by reverent admiration as well as rivalrous envy. The former is known as agape in theology. It is a form of saintly mimesis that is distinct from erotic love or simple affection. The saintly ideals of Caras and Counselors may seem too good to be true, but inspirational models can be sustained for the short duration of camp.

Mimetic desire and cultural blueprints

It might stretch the imagination to suggest that mimesis is a mode of formation similar to embryogenesis. The human embryo seems to self-assemble and becomes a foetus after eight weeks of gestation. Nature has the code or the genome that directs embryogenesis, whilst nurture is the facilitator that can enhance, diminish or interrupt the process. Nature is an internal inheritance, whilst nurture is an external ecology that influences embryonic and foetal formation for good or ill. The peculiarity of mimesis is that the blueprint or form is an external cultural imprint. This is mimetic behaviour, which is effectively an exemplary code that can be incorporated, so that it can then selectively shape our natural abilities. It is easy to comprehend the nature – nurture process of biology, but reversing the direction of influence makes mimesis curiously opaque when it is mimesis of appropriation. Nature is now only the facilitator, whilst culture stipulates the code of apprenticeship or the model of appropriation. In biology, the integrity of the form depends on the accuracy of an internal inheritance. In contrast, the a priori of mimesis is external and visible, but is only effective when incorporated during especially sensitive periods, and even then is subject to interpretation and revision. Mime at other times may distress or amuse, but is not incorporated. Mimesis of appropriation is a subconscious process and occurs when admiration of other persons or objects triggers Eros, our mimetic desire to be like another. This is also the mechanism of role models and mentors:

> Girard argues that desire is ultimately aimed at the mediator's very existence in an attempt – or repeated attempts – to absorb it, to assume it. Metaphysical desire thus describes a desire not for the objects of desire but for the model's uniqueness, spontaneity – his or her 'qualities': Imitative desire is always a desire to be another; Mimetic desire makes us believe we are always on the verge of becoming, self-sufficient through our own transformation into someone else.
>
> (Fleming, 2004:24)

The Eros of mimetic desire is not a constant drive but is especially active in special situations that are effectively halls of mimesis.

Halls of mimesis

Eros is a carte blanche in the newborn and largely shaped and imagined by mimesis of significant others, but mimesis is an interactive process during infancy. Babies are not a passive *tabula rasa*. The mimetic desire of their Eros selectively engages with the world in memorable circumstances. There are halls of mimesis as suggested by Horvath and Szakolczai when we are overwhelmed by a subliminal 'imitative receptivity' and consumed by the identities and the desiring values of others:

> Plato's analysis of Eros as a force that deprives one of one's faculties of distinction and judgement, thus allowing a potentially overwhelming capacity for imitative receptivity to take hold and to drive attempts to possess qualities and constitute identities, but that can at the same time shake up, turn around and elevate.
>
> (Horvath and Szakolczai, 2013:69)

Halls of mimesis begin in the nursery when mimetic desires for the other's toy easily flare into a temper tantrum, unless toddlers are carefully guided by caring adults. Individual squabbles due to little eruptions of mimetic desire are common in preschool children, but contagious violence is not a feature of the nursery. Mimetic desire is immediately apparent in toddlers but becomes subliminal as it floods our grown-up being. Contagious mimesis awaits adolescence and adulthood whether through the spread of fashions amongst teenagers or mimetic violence between gangs and warring nations.

Longings are not our own, but are transmitted in halls of mimesis where we subconsciously appropriate fashionable lifestyles, dress, cuisine and ambitions. These desires seem to be our own but are surreptitiously acquired from others in special situations as unfathomable yearnings that shape our perception and behaviour. Halls of mimesis may vary in size from the school playground to the Nuremberg arena but the coordinating processes are the same: the subliminal absorption of prevailing cultural beliefs, intentions and desires that become taken for granted. We are very careful about choosing situations of formal responsibility for our children whether being cared for in a crèche or taught in a university; but the next generation are also deeply influenced and educated by subterfuge means in halls of mimesis both in the real world and the virtual reality of social media. In halls of mimesis, our guard is down and our mimetic aperture is wide open to the world.

Serious Fun camps are ideal halls of mimesis. Their separation from the real world insulates them from the everyday reality of hospitals and anxious families. The campers in an atmosphere of communitas with their fellows realise that their condition is neither unique nor a handicap. Exhilarating experiences endorsed by revered Masters of Ceremonies open their mimetic aperture to new possibilities. The last days of camp wind down their excitement as they envisage their new-found selves in their home environment. Mimetic social transformations are not risk free, as desires can also be troublesome in the absence of Masters of Ceremonies or the presence of Tricksters. They can generate nasty attributes of envy and violence that can easily get out of hand.

The scapegoat mechanism: antidote to contagious mimetic violence

Mimetic violence triggered by envious greed and rivalry was dangerous to early hominids and threatened extinction of the species (Girard et al., 2007). Innate mechanisms of dominance confines primate aggression to individual confrontations just like toddlers in the nursery, but an enhanced mimetic faculty became contagious in early hominids just as we see in teenagers when their mimetic attention switches from family to peers. Merlin Donald suggests that beneficial mimetic skills in human evolution may have had to co-evolve with the establishment of contagious mimesis. Contagious mimesis could be beneficial as in laughter and crying, but was also dangerous to humanity when linked to aggression. Aggression in our primate forebears was pacified by recognition of the alpha male. In human development, the envy of sparring toddlers also remains confined to individual confrontations. The threat of infectious violence does not appear until the emergence of adolescent gangs. Donald suggests that contagious mimetic violence became a threat to survival in our evolving species when enhanced mimetic skills promoted evolution from *Homo erectus* towards *Homo sapiens*. For Girard, the scapegoat mechanism stayed the violence in a way that eventually led to the foundation of religion and culture. Scapegoats are a terrible profanity as they are random victims external to the affray. Their shocking innocence generates a sacred peace. Peace sanctifies these innocent victims as founders of reconciliation and religious accord.

Myths are censored history cleansed of mimetic violence

According to Girard, the Gods were blamed in ancient lore for human violence; it was a form of self-deception that continued through the ages until the Bible revealed the scapegoat mechanism. Holy institutions that sanctioned transformation of the scapegoat deed into a sacred form misrecognised or censored foregoing internecine violence. For Girard, the ability to read myths and other cultural mechanisms is necessary in order to understand the Bible. Biblical scholars initiated cultural decoding that was a necessary antecedent to the interpretative approach in anthropology and the social sciences. Biblical texts can be read as an *exposé* of the victimage mechanism. Myth and mute have a similar etymology. Myths disguised mimetic violence by cloaking victims in a sacred memory that absolved the perpetrators. The disguise continued until the New Testament identified God with victims rather than the victors. It offered humanity a way of understanding our ancient ethics and morality through a revelation of our muted violent past. A scapegoat victim may be unnecessary if the mechanism was replaced by an ethic of charity and forgiveness as advocated by the New Testament.

Unconstrained mimetic violence does not tally with the mentality of Serious Fun camps, but something like the scapegoat mechanism operates when Caras have finished their training and the first sick children arrive in camp. In Cara interviews, it became clear that there was no rough language when Barretstown was in camp and the signal for a change in style was the arrival of children. The juxtaposition of children and fatal disorders unsettles young adults. The innocence of the children has the power to still profanity and change their caretakers. The Caras say that Barretstown was like a barrack square during training, as they were cursing like troopers, but their language refined spontaneously with the arrival of children to the camp:

> As soon as the kids come through, something happens, you don't use it. And then as soon as they go its 'Jesus', you know…You have a whole new language. It's incredible. At time off we're swearing like dockers.

In a way, children with cancer and leukaemia are scapegoats. They are innocent victims of a potentially fatal disorder, which distinguishes them from other children. Their arrival in the camp changes the behaviour of the Caras. It is a shift from boisterous activity to caring concern. Little did the Caras realise that their concern was about to place them on a pedestal as role models for these children with life-threatening illnesses.

Note

1 Sir William Orpen was a student of personality, temperament, demeanour and style. It was Orpen's business to read the mind's construction in the faces of his sitters. He recognised instantly that the way someone stood, sat or reclined was unique and that tiny movements of a head, hand or foot can be revelatory (Sotheby's catalogue, British and Irish Art London Auction, 22 May 2014).

7 Triangles of desire

Mime artists on a pedestal

Human rituals communicate two classes of information. Self-referential data refer to social status, psychological well-being and physical health, whereas canonical messages are a kind of moral code of verities that cannot be challenged. Self-referential facts are what campers have achieved in the activities and become an index of personal change. The 'Therapeutic Recreation' sequence of challenge, success, reflection and discovery can be regarded as the canon of Barretstown that translates American Camp culture for the rest of the world, and nourishes a desire for joie de vivre modelled by Caras and Counselors. Triangles of desire are a metaphor for the non-linear geometry of desire that can be pathogenic and prone to rivalry when subject and model are in the same social space; but salutogenic during Serious Fun experiences as campers and counselors are in the different kingdoms of the sick and the well.

> Mimetic desire is what makes us human, what makes possible for us the breakout from routinely animalistic appetites, and constructs our own, albeit inevitably unstable, identities. It is this very mobility of desire, its mimetic nature, and this very instability of our identities, that makes us capable of adaptation.
>
> René Girard (*Evolution and Conversion,* 2007)

Theorists emphasise that Masters of Ceremonies are the important source of social order in liminal situations. Novices stripped of their former identity through various humiliations in traditional rites of passage need Masters of Ceremonies. They are vulnerable to being led astray by tricksters before being tested for their transformation to an elevated status (Horvath and Thomassen, 2008). Masters of Ceremonies provide guidance into the canon of traditional tribal verities, while novices participate in challenging self-referential activities (Rappaport, 1999). Rappaport's canon is a kind of subliminal cultural ethos, whilst self-referential activities by novices are evidence of their worthiness for promotion. Self-referential activities are very evident in Serious Fun campers whether in high ropes or theatrical performances, but the canon is less obvious. The essence of Serious Fun camps is that Counselors and Caras are models of canonical behaviour that embodies an ideal and possibility of health and well-being. They are both the guardians of the children and a visible ethos of wholesome lifestyles that live on in the campers as noted by a Cara:

> I wouldn't have thought we were having such a big effect on children until I spoke to a former camper at the ten-year anniversary. He was at the gala ball and he saw two of his former Caras across the room; and it took him the entire night to build up the courage and go over and speak to them. Because since he was ten or eleven, he held them in such a high regard that he would always remember back on his time in Barretstown and remember such and such did this and why they were amazing. They obviously had such a huge impact on his life, that I am sure that the two of them had no idea that they had done that.

They can be impeccable role models when inspired by seriously ill children for the short duration of the camp. The role that they model is not precise. It is more an intimation of possibility – a *weltanschauung* and a way of being in the world. The children's experiences of camp are not just a dream come true but a reinvigorating salutogenic world view. The world becomes meaningful, it can be understood and coped with despite the tribulations of serious life-threatening illnesses.

Triangles of mimetic desire

From Girard's perspective, mimetic desire has a triangular form composed by the subject and the object of desire at the base and the model as a mediator at the apex (Girard, 1996b). The subject longs for objects and personal qualities through a third party. The model or mediator is an apparently superior being that sets standards. The subject desires valuables that are attributes or objects belonging to exemplary models in a social milieu of mimetic longing. Attributes and objects are seen as desirable because they are deemed valuable by esteemed others. It is an opaque process as the dials of mimetic desire are extrinsic to the self and rotated by inappreciable cultural forces. It is a masked agency. Girard's concern was for what he called internal mimesis, but proximal mimesis may be a better term: proximal in the sense of being a socially available temptation. He was also aware of an alternative external or a distal relationship of desire.

The shape of the triangle

The triangle can be a responsive metaphor (Figure 7.1) for the geometry of desire, as the shape of the triangle reflects the type of relationship between the subject and the mediator. Close relationships of mimetic desire in the same social space can be reflected as an equilateral triangle. The proximity of the subject and the mediating model exposes the latter to the lure of reciprocal desire. The mediator may now experience Eros via the subject's desire. They both desire the same object. The proximal model is close enough to the subject in terms of social status, time and reality that interaction can generate envy and rivalry. Relationships between subject and model may initially be one sided, but eventually a competitive edge tends to be reciprocated. The object of desire may become incidental to a developing rivalry as the relationship becomes increasingly antagonistic and destructive. Social interaction adopts a tangible competitive edge that is apparent to all in the same realm. Rivalry can spiral to communal intra-species violence – the great problem of humanity, but its mimetic quality is invariably misrecognised. Internal mimetic desire contains a positive and negative double bind: the positive yearns for the socially desirable and the negative demands revenge. This is what Girard described as internal mimesis. The Girardian subject embroiled in a social field of internal mimesis misinterprets beliefs and values that shape intentionality. The scene is set for 'monstrous doubling' as the pendulum of desire shifts to jealousy between the subject and the model. Rivalry foments desire in both subject and model, so that the value of the desired object may spiral beyond reason provoking a situation of 'monstrous doubles'. In monstrous doubles, the subject and the model become mirror images of one another as in an arms race, so that violence may spiral beyond available social controls. Eros unleashes subconscious desires in both the subject and the model, which can escalate towards envious rivalry and physical violence. This pathogenic relationship is contagious and may recruit bystanders into the fray. In monstrous doubles, the subject and the model become mirror images of one another as in an arms race when the potential for aggression may increase beyond common sense and judicial controls. The initial trigger of mimetic desire may even be forgotten as violence spirals beyond available social constraints with apocalyptic consequences.

The Cara–camper mimetic relationship in Barretstown does not contain a whit of envy or rivalry. The beneficial effect of salutogenic desires mediated by the Cara as a model can be explained by Girard's triangle of external mimesis or what can be called distal mimesis in a terminology of social anatomy. The hallowed relationships of distal mimesis between subjects and revered mediators are more spiritual than temporal. Christian doctrine advised adherents to imitate the lives of the saints. The shape of imitation in distal mimesis changes to an isosceles triangle (Figure 7.1) as the social distance extends to a heavenly space. Caras and Counselors in an atmosphere of Serious Fun provide seriously ill children with a template for salutogenesis in the real world. It is effectively a one-way relationship as the saintly mediator at the apex of the triangle is blissfully unaware of the subject's adulation. There is no risk of 'monstrous doubles' as subjects and mediators operate in different realms. Counselors and the children effectively exist in Susan Sontag's different kingdoms of the sick and the well in Serious Fun camps (Sontag, 1991). They live in separate social spaces that cannot be bridged. The divide

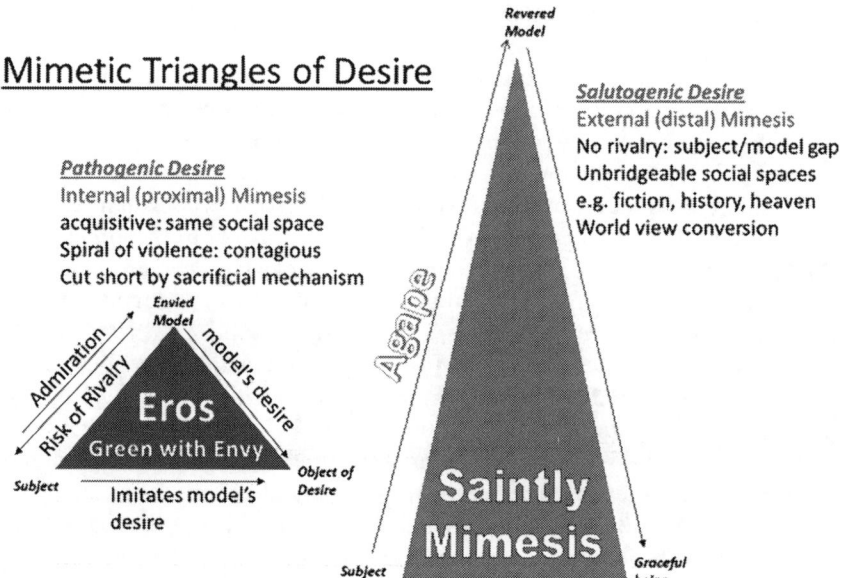

Figure 7.1 The triangle as a metaphor. The triangle, of course, is nothing but a metaphor that expresses the non-linear geometry of desire, a structural model
that changes in shape and size according to the distance between the mediator and the imitator. It has no existence in reality (Merrill, 2013:13).

ensures a salutogenic relationship between sick children and their healthy
mentors. The children's desire to be like their mentors can be imagined as an
isosceles triangle. The nature of Eros changes as well and is better expressed
by the theological term of Agape (spellbound, Christian love). In the figure,
the shape of the triangles illustrates the spectrum of desire that ranges from
the immediacy of Eros in internal mimesis to revered Agape that is external
and transcendent. The latter relationship works in Serious Fun camps but
has come under scrutiny elsewhere since the egalitarian ideals of modernity
challenges the hierarchy of exemplary models.

Modernity and exemplary models

The egalitarian ideal of modernity poses a problem for those advocating
external mimesis as the way to reform identities. Modernity is hostile to
traditional authority and is reticent about any kind of deference towards distinction. Exemplary models are in short supply since the Enlightenment. The
valorisation of equality has the paradoxical effect of engendering romantic
individualism independent of social hierarchy. Quests for role models since
the Enlightenment redirect individuals towards an internal personal authenticity. Plumbing psychological depths for an authentic self without a model

as guide is a recipe for hollow men. Authentic selves cannot be constituted without a suitable model. Lost souls grappling in vain for internal guidance in a state of uncertainty is a terrifying situation. It is the locus of the great angst of the twentieth century. The demand for equality undermines reliable models, so the mimetic quest for suitable mentors is more likely to fail in modernity. Equality discourages distinction and quality – the hallmarks of exemplary models. Serious Fun camps are a modern exception in that their founding father was a Hollywood star; their ultra-modern godparents were the *avant-garde* of clinical research in Paediatric Oncology; they happened in the informal and mainly egalitarian cultures of the late twentieth century in the Western World; nevertheless, Caras and Counselors are revered by campers in the special space–time capsules that are Serious Fun camps. They are Carers and Masters of Ceremonies and as such are ideal salutogenic models. The structure of camp facilitates transient liminality, which opens campers to the canonical lifestyle values of their exemplary models. Caras and Counselors can sustain their role as inspirational models to seriously ill children for the short duration of camp.

Eros, Agape and Philia

Human desires are often capricious until they are guided by another person:

> Once basic needs are satisfied, humans remain governed by intense yearning, which is at first uncertain about which objects to desire.
>
> (Palaver, 2013:35)

In mimetic triangles, subjects long for an object through a third party. This book suggests that the mimetic relationship between Camper and Counselor in Serious Fun camps is like that of Agape between disciple and sage. In the camp, the Caras and Counselors are models of health whose apparent superior being sets admired lifestyles mimed subconsciously by campers. It is a form of adulation or Agape encouraged in the past by Lives of the Saints. In contrast, mimetic Eros covets goods and valuables of others: the wives and goods of the ninth and tenth commandments, which the ancients understood as dangerous to peaceful co-existence. Envied persons set desired standards and act as rivals in a social milieu of mimetic longing. What seems to be a personal fancy has instead been hankered after by subconsciously imitating the aspirations of others. It is an opaque process as the dials of mimetic desire are extrinsic to the self and operated by inapparent cultural forces. The excitement and reverence of Agape in the campers needs to be grounded before leaving towards Philia (Keohane and Cuhling, 2014): the Philia that loves and respects the ancient humane institutions of home, family and community before returning to the more mundane interactions of the real world. Mimetic desire has a masked agency, although material desires that conflict with the commandments are easier to recognise than spiritual identification with the ethos of revered mentors. Observations and interviews in different Serious Fun camps suggest that the Association inspired by Paul Newman has managed to reproduce ancient ways of ritual change in the mentality of seriously ill children. The process can be theorised as a mimetic mentoring relationship favouring Agape rather than Eros that can be grounded towards Philia in the 'real world'.

Mimetic Eros: *Dia agus Diabhal* (God and the devil)

> There is a startling difference between the attractive goodness and beauty that gathers people together, one by one, in saintly discipleship and the evil that spreads division through the masses.
>
> (Paul Ricoeur, 1998, cited in Astell, 2004:116)

Mimetic human desire can be a source of greed, envy and violence, but also an inspiration for 'attractive goodness and beauty' in different circumstances. God and the devil are two sides of the same mimetic coin acknowledged *as Gaeilge* by the close pronunciations of *Dia* and *Diabhal*. Eros is a wild card in liminal situations and has the power to propel participants towards either pole of the mimetic coin. According to Hamerton-Kelly (1992), Eros and Agape are extremes of mimetic human desire – Eros reflecting a disposition towards acquisition and conflict – whereas the desire of Agape is gracious and generous; in other words, two forms of the same basic human propensity, one alienated and the other integrated. This book takes Eros as the generic form of human desire that when undisciplined can be a source of greed, envy and violence or a disciplined inspiration for 'attractive goodness and beauty' when transfigured to Agape. Eros is desire deformed by acquisitive and conflictual mimesis; Agape is desire reformed by gracious and generous mimetic behaviour. Both generous and conflictual mimetic impulses are always mediated through a model, so that, for Girard (1996b), mimesis has triangular forms as illustrated above.

An Diabhal: the devil and the gift relation

There was deep shock when *The Star* (Irish edition August 31st, 2006) published news of the arrest of the camp director of Barretstown for downloading child pornography. He had been instantly fired from Barretstown when this was discovered through broadband monitoring. Emails from Barretstown administration were sent to all volunteer staff and parents indicating that there was no evidence that the children had been harmed in any way. The story then died. It did not appear on the national broadsheets or any other media. The response of the press with a single exception had been respectful and recognised that there will be breaches in screening despite careful vigilance. An earlier interview with the disgraced camp director gave excellent insight into the workings of the camp, and a more insightful analysis on the role of professional and volunteer staff than previous interviews with the administrative staff. A senior staff member subsequently commented:

> There was a general disbelief because the person in question was very good at what he did. And very pleasant, sociable all of the things, you know, on face value, yes what you saw was very pleasant. It caused me great distress in how could that be and the other piece that I found very interesting was a lot of them said we never saw anything... now if you want to be in this business, this is part and parcel of it, but it is the darker side. But it exists and it's there. It did shake them up. In a peculiar way afterwards, the following camp made them even more determined to continue to do the work. This place is greater than the individual. And all of the support staff they all stepped up and took over and ran the rest of the summer and ran it very well.

At first sight, he was a Trickster figure, but there was no suggestion that he had any corrupting influence in the camp. In anthropological literature, the liminal phases in rites of passage are often endangered by the presence of Tricksters. The spirit of Tricksters, born of chaos and disruption intrinsic to transformative processes, can derail the meaning-giving and identity-building process. The Trickster causes trouble by corrupting the gift relation. The gift relation was effectively interrupted for children attending the leukaemia clinic in Cork. The Social Worker there felt that it was her responsibility to warn parents of a danger in Barretstown and it took time to restore the parents' confidence in the camp. This happened through word of mouth rather than any policy directives. The integrity and sustainability of Barretstown was undoubtedly threatened, but there was also the remarkable response of the media. The media would usually treat such an instance as a cynical opportunity for lurid reporting, but instead there was uncharacteristic restraint, evidence of the prevailing power of respect surrounding Barretstown.

Mol an Óige agus Tiocfaidh Siad (praise the young and they will flourish)

The violence of childhood cancer establishes a need for a social response that can be understood as part of the sacrificial mechanism. The sacrificial mechanism is a system that draws attention to the outrage of unfair victimisation and changes attitudes. In this case, children with life-threatening illnesses inspire the establishment of Serious Fun camps. Serious Fun camp experiences exclude the vicious circle of mimetic rivalry because the model in the desiring triangle is too distal from the subject. From the sick child's perspective, the Counselors are in a different realm. The dialectic between the two cannot be a vicious spiral of envy. Their distinctive kingdoms of sickness and health ensure a virtuous circle of inspiration. Mimetic friendships between mentors and apprentices are based on mutual admiration at different levels of being. Serious fun is the elixir of camp that sets an atmosphere of wonderland. Serious play is a virtuous circle where praise and encouragement from esteemed Caras relives the old Irish saying: *mol an óige agus tiocfaidh siad* – praise the young and they will flourish.

Types of social space and mediated desire of Eros and Agape

The equilateral triangle illustrates mediated desire between denizens in the same social space. Mediated desire sets the scene for potentially violent relationships between the envious subject and the mediator. The original object of jealousy may be forgotten in a spiral of violence, which Girard called internal mimesis. Proximal mimesis envisaged as an equilateral triangle is a suitable alternative, as the subject and the mediator need to be in the same social space. The proximal model is close enough to generate envy and rivalry. Initial relationships between the subject and the model may be one sided, but eventually a competitive edge emerges. The object of desire may become incidental to a developing rivalry. In these circumstances, the relationship between the subject and the model becomes increasingly antagonistic and destructive. Rivalry can spiral to communal intra-species violence – the great problem of humanity. For Girard, this was an internally mediated desire, whereby lack of distance (spatial, temporal or spiritual) between the model and the subject led to risks of mimetic conflict. A tangible competitive edge to social interaction between the subject and the model becomes apparent to all in the same realm, but its mimetic quality is invariably misrecognised. The potential for conflict arises because near-perfect imitation will result in the subject trying to displace the model.

The Cara/Counselor and camper relationships in Serious Fun experiences do not contain a hint of jealousy. The beneficial effect of the camper's desire can be explained through Girard's triangle of external mimesis. This form of mimetic relationship was not explored in depth by Girard, but he recognised an alternative mimetic relationship that was non-violent. Campers as subjects may still relate to revered models as mediators of desire in a different realm that can be envisaged as an isosceles triangle with a distal apex. The context of the separate realm may be historical, spiritual, fictional or healthful, but the mediators are detached from the everyday reality of the subjects. The different realm creates a gap between the model and the subject, so that the relationship is one sided. Unequal relationships cannot arouse mediators, so there is no question of rivalry or envy. The subject is in thrall to the mediator, but the latter is blissfully unaware of adulation and admiration. The charismatic model transforms the perceptual field of the subject creating a new reality. A Cara recalls that the first question of returning campers was whether their Caras were still in Barretstown:

> I had a family last week who had been here last year and their first question was are A and M still here? They knew exactly who their two Caras were, you could even see the attachment that grew.

Desire is a diverse phenomenon that can be triggered by envy or respect. Mediated desire is strangely opaque to society and can be a deeply subconscious internal motivation. The process tends to remain invisible to the subject even when it is an evident external ambition. Girard describes metaphysical desire as an attraction to or a fascination with figures that signify a fullness of being. It is a desire for the model's qualities. It occurs in the kind of scenario that 'men will become gods for each other' as when an appropriate mediator will be able to fill a felt lack.

Mimetic innovation and the gift relationship

The sacred time-out-of-time atmosphere of Serious Fun camps may be in keeping with the sacrificial mechanism. There is an element of the sacred in Serious Fun camps. Sick children play in superb facilities despite the profanity of life-threatening illnesses. Serious Fun camps are not only a transient sanctuary for children who have spent too much of their young lives in hospital, but are also a place where they can be liberated from a sense of social exclusion. An element of the sacred arose in group interviews with Caras and was reiterated in other Serious Fun camps. The Caras discussed the question of religion together:

> 'Somebody asked me is it a Catholic thing? And I said no, religion is not really part of it'. 'everyone is here for one thing to help the children'. 'It's just shared experiences. It's like a new religion'. 'It's just real people on the ground and what they have been through'. 'It's not focused on are you Muslim, Buddhist, Christian? It's focused more on people'.

There is also a mimetic sociability amongst the Caras and Counselors maintained by gift relationships:

> I also think we see our job as one game. Like I don't just walk territory and say if you don't get yours done, I don't care – mine's done and I'm going to finish it quick and sit down here and have a cup of tea. It's like the whole thing is one job. So if you need help picking up your side or I need help picking up my side, you jump in and do that. We carry the ball together instead of lots of little balls.

The Caras have a job, and they summarised it with a quote from 'The Godfather':

> 'this is the business we have chosen'. The staff are on the same wave length. We all have a common goal to make the kids happy and make sure they have fun. We are not doing this for the money. We are not doing this for the time off. The reward is actually the children and the response you get from them'.

Theoretical summary

All Serious Fun camps founded by Paul Newman have a rite of passage space–time structure as first described by Arnold van Gennep in 1908, but not published in English until 1960. Profane and sacred worlds were distinct in ancient and tribal worlds and had to be linked by a formal ritual passage. Rites of passage have a tripartite structure with stages of separation, transition and re-integration. Serious Fun camps manage the children's separation from their real world of hospital, family and social media in a way that is remarkably complete. Victor Turner emphasised the sense of liminality in the transitional stage when rules are in abeyance, conventions relaxed and passengers tested in a communal frame. This risky situation requires Masters of Ceremonies to oversee the process. Common challenging experiences generate feelings of communitas – a bonding fellowship of shared possibilities and change in the air. Rituals coordinate natural change to suit the social world. Status change is the traditional form of social transformation in these transient passages, but status elevation did not match the type of transformation noted in these seriously ill children. Something else changed, which can be understood in terms of mimesis.

Merlin Donald (1991) has suggested that our prelingual ancestors communicated in mimetic cultures. Mimes unlike symbols are concrete and confined to the present. They may have been the communication media that prefigured the beginning of abstract speech as replayed in early childhood development. Mimetic communication is often ambiguous, humorous and sly but is only the tip of the iceberg. Mimesis is largely subconscious and coordinates transmission of cultural lifestyles as seems to happen in camp. Caras and Counselors are Masters of Ceremonies in Serious Fun rites of passage but are also the campers' instrument of change. Girard's theories of external mimesis and the sacrificial mechanism provide suitable concepts for understanding the process. Serious Fun camps support subconscious mimetic transformations of seriously ill children towards a healthful world view exemplified by their Caras and Counselors as models for external mediation.

The structural situation of the sick child at the Serious Fun camp can be understood in terms of violence and the sacrificial mechanism. Childhood cancer or leukaemia can be understood as a random act of natural violence on innocent victims. The presence of very ill children in the camps operates the sacrificial mechanism, so that, in a Girardian sense, their innocent victimhood generates a sacred space. The ground becomes sacred and the children are venerated – they are as Anthropologists say effectively in worship. Girard's reading of the New Testament recognises the transformation from polytheism to monotheism: from those Gods of violence who sanctified bullies, to the God of victims who revealed their innocence. The Christian world offered a lens from the victim's perspective. That is the perspective to view the special position of ill children in the liminal world of camp. It sets the scene for their transformation.

The rite of passage space–time structure of transient liminality produces spontaneous communitas that effectively undifferentiates the children. They shed their Royal Stigma, the social baggage of chronic illness. They are liberated from a marginal position in society. They open a mimetic window to their soul. Their undifferentiated state risks being led astray, but they can be re-orientated by focussed mimetic desire on a suitable external image. Mimetic desire seeks an object, a style or an attitude that is embodied in an admired model. In external mimesis, the model cannot be a rival because their image is from an unattainable realm. The intense Platonic relationship between Caras and campers permits external mimetic transformations. The Caras and Counselors have a crucial role. The children are not a poor reflection of their mentors but are inspired by their Caras. It is a process of sanctification in the sense of being made whole. The Caras may only be a few years older than teenage campers, yet the psychological gap between them is enormous as Caras embody an ideal of health and ability that appears elusive and unattainable to the campers. The gap between Caras as external models and the children as subjects can be mediated by play.

Huizinga (1955) has drawn our attention to a playful mode of being that is fundamental to humanity. Play is the chief mode of social interaction in Serious Fun camps dominated by an exhilarating subjunctive mood. The indicative moods of hospital routines are forgotten. The camp world is protected, and it has a play style of friendly public performances which can only be sustained in situations that are totally separate from mundane evaluations. A caring atmosphere can gently interrogate the campers' axiology with the potential to generate new values and ethical codes that may only become apparent after re-integration to society. Moments of ludic liminality have powers of transformation akin to wreaths of wild olives awarded to ancient Greek Olympians. The symbolic wreath is sufficient for communal recognition. At a more personal level in the camp, the wreath equivalent abstracts to an approving glance, a smile or a word of encouragement provided by respected mentors together with recognition of personal achievements by fellow campers. The ludic mentality is not without risk as tricksters can easily corrupt and even further isolate the socially stricken. The distinction between counterfeit and genuine mimesis is crucial as children can be easily led astray in liminal situations.

8   The magi

Three wise men bearing gifts

Most researchers beaver within a mould of practice but a few are exceptional and break the mould. The three men mentioned here contributed to the great breakthrough in Paediatric Oncology in the latter half of the twentieth century that led to medical and social revolutions in the care of children with life threatening illnesses. It took twenty years to establish the principles of care in the management of acute lymphoblastic leukaemia in children, whereas the social revolution of care was an accidental by-product of philanthropy. It is the difference between cognition and recognition. Medical cognition requires theories that can be slowly tested in clinical trials whereas breakthroughs in social care are often accidental assemblies of a care pattern that are subsequently recognised as beneficial.

> The Indian giver understood a cardinal property of the gift: whatever we have been given is supposed to be given away again not kept.
>
> *Lewis Hyde*: The Gift

The Indian giver as part of a gift economy was misunderstood by the white man and his market economy. Talent should be shared and not hoarded as did the three wise men noted here. The etymology of Prophecy suggests a gift for interpreting the will of God. Max Weber wrote on the importance of Prophecy in times of stress and the role Prophets played in redirecting humanity to a better place. It seems anachronistic nowadays to think in terms of Prophets and Prophecy, but Prophets as ideal types from old time religions suggest how societies can respond to pitiless events that challenge a secular world.

Ideal types

Weber's 'ideal type' is an example of either a social style of behaviour (for example, a Prophet) or a social process (for example, a Prophecy) from history that may assist understanding of real contemporary situations. It is a confusing term as Weber's types are not ideal in the sense of being the best, but are more a sharp outline of peculiarities that emphasise distinguishing characteristics of social types. They are like a cartoon in which key features and characteristics are emphasised as a memorable type. We subconsciously use ideal types all the time to facilitate our engagement with the world as a summary of people and events. A photograph taken by Jimmy Sime before the annual cricket game between Eton and Harrow in 1937 is a classic example of ideal types. His front-page picture of two types of schoolboy labelled 'Toffs and Toughs' seemed to illustrate the class divide in pre-war Britain. The imperious de-meanour of the 'Toffs' contrasted with the cheeky faces of the 'Toughs'. As it turned out, the 'Toffs' life was tragic, whereas the 'Toughs' had happy and fulfilling biographies. The photo portrayed an 'ideal type' of class division in England, whereas subsequent life experiences of the boys were unrelated to their 'ideal type'.[1] Ideal types are a short-hand attempt to rationalise and therefore understand observed social processes and behaviours. Natural sci-entists construct biological models that can replicate findings of experimental data. Social scientists use 'ideal-type' examples from historical models to il-luminate events and experiences in our contemporary world.

Magicians, Priests and Prophets

Weber (1978) contrasted three religious 'ideal types' from ancient history beginning with the temporary charisma of the Magician, when he plied his magic from a rural base. The Priest was Weber's second type. His Priesthood had an urban base and Priests unlike the Magician were part of the ruling authority. A Prophet on the other hand had a vocation inspired by revelation. His power related to personal charisma, which could instigate revolutionary social change. Prophets grasped a singular understanding of crises that could suggest meaningful solutions. Magicians and Priests were a constant presence in ancient societies, whereas Prophets only appeared during times of instabil-ity. Priests and Prophets were often at loggerheads as Prophets were hostile to sacrifice and other customs promoted by Priests to placate prevailing God-heads. Solutions offered by Prophets in times of trouble required confron-tation with the prevailing order. Weber distinguished two types of Prophet depending on how they responded to revelations. Exemplary Prophets man-ifested their insight through a style of behaviour that set an example to fol-lowers. Ethical Prophets on the other hand were inspired to spread a message. The perceived veracity of their revelation depended on genuine personal charisma. The emphasis was on their revelatory insight rather than their con-duct. The truthfulness of the message was apparent through their authentic bearing. In ancient history, Prophets appeared in times of distress variously called times of trouble (Toynbee), the axial age (Jaspers, Eisenstadt), the ecu-menic age (Voegelin), liminal periods (Szakolczai) and a *sattelzeit* (Koselleck) (Szakolczai, 2003b:30). These different descriptions probably depended on the type of social organisation in disarray. Clearly unstable times such as the axial age and ecumenic age refer to slow tectonic plate social change in vast empires that is imperceptible in the everyday, even though eventual social collapse like the fall of Rome may occur suddenly. On the other hand, times of trouble may be more apt for relatively brief social crises that are local and do not require a historical perspective.

Disruptive family experiences because of life-threatening illness in their children such as childhood cancer may be better understood as 'times of trouble' or 'liminal periods'. This kind of devastation may need intervention from latter-day Prophets in order to divine alternative answers to present-day turmoil. The whole process of cancer diagnosis and treatment in children is a recipe for social disruption. Cancer protocols for children may upset family cohesion through a necessity for prolonged hospitalisation away from home with associated risks of sibling neglect, parental unemployment and economic hardship.

Weber's religious 'ideal types' in health and illness

Weber's religious types – the Magician, the Priest and the Prophet – may assist our understanding of contemporary social processes in the domain of health and illness. The purveyors of alternative medicine have a role that is not too different from Magicians. Alternative practitioners like Magicians are outside the mainstream of accepted medical practice. They largely ply their trade in the realm of the placebo effect. The placebo effect is an important facet of treatment, but clinical therapeutics tend to dismiss its effect as a troublesome intrusion when measuring drug efficacy. Modern medical establishments claim authority based on scientific methods. They are a Priesthood with their own hierarchy. They have powerful rituals that are effective in combating most physical disorders, even if they are less competent in matters of social distress. The authority of medical practice in any society depends on its efficacy. New health issues and complications may undermine the prevailing medical wisdom. Latter day Prophets may then emerge to challenge the system as inadequate and propose alternative practices. In the latter half of the twentieth century, wise men emerged to challenge the prevailing caring systems of seriously ill children. Donald Pinkel, Danny Thomas and Paul Newman were inspirational leaders with a calling, and each in their own way transformed the care of children with life-threatening illnesses.

Donald Pinkel

Paediatricians in the 1950s regarded a career in childhood cancers as misguided. Treatment failures imbued these malignancies with a fatalistic aura. At that time, Donald Pinkel expressed his desire as a young Paediatrician to focus on paediatric cancer research. He was strongly advised by his head of department against specialisation in childhood cancer so as not to throw away his career in a therapeutic *cul-de-sac*. The grim reaper oversaw conditions like acute leukaemia. Sydney Farber's research was regarded as a false dawn. Most Paediatricians judged experimental research on children with malignancies as unacceptable and only a way of prolonging suffering. Despite that advice, Pinkel spent time with the Clinical Cancer Investigators at the National Cancer Institute. He took up the position of Founding Director at St. Jude's Children's Hospital in

1961. In St. Jude's, Pinkel became an inspirational leader in the emerging specialty of Paediatric Oncology. Although Donald Pinkel had spent some time as a research fellow in Farber's department, his basic training was that of a Paediatrician. Cancer and leukaemia were fearful diagnoses for young Paediatricians in the 1950s as it was then the commonest cause of death in children over a year old. Even as a medical student, Donald Pinkel was drawn towards this cause of heartbreak. He had a deep personal understanding of severe chronic illness as he caught polio from his young patients whilst a paediatric resident. He nearly died of respiratory failure. His rehabilitation was slow. Even at the height of his fame, he still bore traces of polio in 1972, when invited to London to give the Annual Leukaemia Research Fund lecture. He had a warm, unassuming presence, but walked with a slight limp. By that time, Pinkel had been Founding Director of St. Jude's Children's Hospital, Memphis, Tennessee, for ten years. Since 1962, he and his colleagues had imagined necessary principles to cure half of children presenting with acute lymphoblastic leukaemia. Donald Pinkel would be the last person to think of himself as a Prophet, but he fulfilled Weber's criteria of having a vocation, a visionary revelation and charismatic leadership that achieved a paradigm revolution in the care of children with cancer. Paediatric Oncology emerged from its experimental origins to become an effective, exciting and challenging subspecialty.

Danny Thomas

One could say that Danny Thomas and Donald Pinkel are an unlikely pair of latter day Prophets, but their separate visions aligned in St. Jude's Children's Research Hospital. Danny Thomas made a vow as a young starving actor that he would build a shrine to St Jude, the patron saint of hopeless causes, if he could find showtime success. His vision was that 'no children should die at the dawn of life'. It was an extravagant supplication for an unemployed entertainer. Danny Thomas was born in Michigan to Lebanese Maronite Catholic immigrants in 1912. He was one of ten children and christened Amos Muzyad Yakhoob. He did not forget St Jude after he became a very successful television personality and changed his name to Danny Thomas. He formed a consortium of business interests in the 1950s to help fund his ambition. Eventually, they would build a magnificent shrine to St Jude in Memphis, Tennessee, with the guidance of Cardinal Stritch, spiritual mentor to Danny Thomas. St. Jude's Children's Research Hospital opened in 1962 with Donald Pinkel as its founding director. The vision of Danny Thomas bordered on hubris, but it was the beginning of realistic hopes of a cure for children with cancer at the dawn of life.

Paediatric Oncology: a paradigm shift in child health

Prophets from religious worlds attribute visions to revelations from heavenly beings; but Prophecy is not confined to solutions from the spiritual realm. Research scientists also need inspiration. Thomas Kuhn (1996) observed two kinds of research: problem solving within an accepted paradigm and paradigm revolutions, which changed the rules of research. The latter are exceptional as most research is a slow assembly of knowledge within an accepted scientific paradigm. The emergence of Paediatric Oncology may seem to have been a problem-solving answer to treatment of childhood cancers, but it was a paradigm revolution as it changed the rules of paediatric therapeutics and eventually priorities governing social care of sick children. This chapter focusses on three latter day Prophets, whose inspirations led medical and social revolutions in the care of children with life-threatening illnesses. The treatment breakthrough in childhood acute leukaemia became the standard example of best practice for all clinical trials in cancer. Experimental chemotherapy by Sydney Farber and other Haematologists was a necessary prelude to the masterful systematic studies of Pinkel and colleagues. They showed through several innovations in St. Jude's Children's Research Hospital that it was possible to cure acute lymphoblastic leukaemia. Sydney Farber et al (1948) had tried cytotoxic drugs one after the other in a series, pushing doses of each drug until the leukaemia was visibly eradicated under the microscope or the toxic side effects were too harsh. Initial optimism was replaced by disillusionment as the children died of relapse or drug toxicity. Pinkel had learned from his colleagues in the National Cancer Institute that combination chemotherapy was more effective in prolonging remissions and less toxic than maximal doses of single drugs. Pinkel and colleagues combined cytotoxic drugs that had different side effects, so that more treatment could be easily given. They recognised that obtaining a remission was inadequate and instituted maintenance treatment, with an early phase of intensification after initial remission induction. Children survived for longer, but late relapses in the Central Nervous System became a problem. Evidently leukaemia cells can seed the spinal fluid around the time of diagnosis. These cells were effectively insulated from combination chemotherapy because the blood–brain barrier prevented cytotoxic drugs gaining access to the cerebro-spinal fluid. In healthy children, the blood–brain barrier is useful as it protects the central nervous system from circulating noxious agents. The blood–brain barrier was a hindrance to a cure in children with leukaemia as it prevented curative cytotoxic drugs from reaching the brain. The central nervous system was effectively a sanctuary site as leukaemia cells could still proliferate there despite effective chemotherapy for the rest of the body. Sanctuary sites emerged as a source of relapse, so the St Jude protocols instituted separate treatment of the brain at the beginning of treatment to prevent later relapse in the central nervous system. These innovations were the basis of the first reliable cures in the treatment of acute lymphoblastic leukaemia in children. These fundamental discoveries changed the attitude of Paediatricians towards innovative treatment of malignancies. It was a revolutionary change in the rules of medical practice. Children could now be at the forefront of clinical research with

Paediatric Oncology as a prime example. The experience of acute child-hood leukaemia changed from suffering a devastating illness with a death sentence to suffering from the consequences of treatment that might include the side effects of drugs and radiotherapy, but also existential psychological worries about social exclusion. It took another twenty years more before a third Prophet emerged to imagine Serious Fun camps that were a revolution in the social care of children with life-threatening disorders.

Paul Newman

The argument for a social revolution in care is the same as that for a medical revolution. Newman was an ethical Prophet, distinguished by charisma, a personal call and a revelation. Ethical Prophets propose fundamental breaks in prevailing conventions and proclaim, an insight that challenges the ruling authority. His followers were aware that he had a vocation[2] 'he was possessed by the camp spirit'. Furthermore, he had a message: 'I have this idea and you have got to listen'. His idea was simple, but also a fundamental break in estab-lished medical wisdom. His revelation was that camping should be available for children with life-threatening illnesses. He divined that the problems of chronic severe childhood illnesses could be ameliorated by camp experiences. His initial intuition was that these children would benefit from a holiday away from the hospital gaze. 'I don't think he know the trajectory of this when he started'. He certainly challenged authority 'and people kept saying you can't do it because of this. And he'd say no, no, no'.

It is difficult to know whether Paul Newman should be regarded as a Ma-gician or a Prophet, but perhaps he was both. After all, in ancient religions, Prophets emerged from Magicians and not from the Priesthood. At first sight, Newman seems an unlikely Prophet, as he was a cinema icon who seemed to relish antihero roles. Those of the correct vintage will remember him in roles such as *The Hustler, Somebody Up There Likes me* and *Butch Cassidy and the Sundance Kid*. He was happiest when racing fast cars. He was a contemporary of Marlon Brando and James Dean (most famous for *Rebel Without a Cause*). They were members of the method generation in the 1950s that immersed themselves in their roles. Both Dean and Brando rapidly rose to fame. Their ends were less glamorous: Dean died aged twenty-four in a car crash, whilst Brando had a long and quarrelsome relationship with Hollywood until his death aged 80. All three actors were megastars, but Newman managed to separate Hollywood fame from his family life.

The death of Newman's eldest son of three children from his first marriage left him bereft. It is tempting to apply this biographical experience to his sub-sequent role as a founder of Hole in the Wall, the first Serious Fun camp, but ethical Prophets have an innate quality, which is an ability to diagnose flaws in the zeitgeist. Biographical circumstances – the conditions of emergence – shape the Prophecy, but not the Prophet. Behind the cinema roles, he was different. The icon from *Butch Cassidy and the Sundance Kid* was anything but Hollywood. He was a step up from James Dean as he was a rebel with a cause. The fleeting relationships of the film set and Los Angeles were not for him. For first and foremost, Paul Newman was a family man and remained happily married to his second wife for fifty years. The Newman family lived in Connecticut, not too far from the Hole in the Wall Camp, the first Serious Fun camp in Ashford. The antihero mask disguised his mission; for he was a Prophet, a visionary who saw solutions to the plight of a relatively new phenomenon in the 1980s – chronic severe illness in children – perhaps best exemplified by childhood cancer and leukaemia.

Newman was regarded as a celebrity philanthropist in Barretstown, the Irish Serious Fun camp. It was different in Hole in the Wall, the Connecticut camp, where the fact that he was a generous philanthropist was almost incidental. The staff in the Hole in the Wall Gang Camp knew him well as he was a frequent visitor and sat on various committees. He was dying in 2008, when I visited the Hole in the Wall Gang Camp, and any inquiries about him at that time were met with a protective response. Nobody wanted prying eyes on a man that they clearly loved and respected. Charisma may be inborn and that seems to have been the case with Newman. He always described himself as lucky. He was spoken of with reverence by those who knew him well. His colleagues, his fan base and even the media did not have a bad word to say about him.

In the 1980s, children with cancer and leukaemia were becoming more visible in the community. Paul Newman became convinced that a camping experience would be beneficial for these children. Maybe it was because Newman was an instinctive philanthropist in search of a cause, but he never answered queries as to why he adopted children with cancer as beneficiaries of his obsession. His relentless pursuit of enabling camp for seriously ill children was more in keeping with a visionary ethical Prophet. Newman repeatedly challenged the prevailing therapeutic wisdom. The medical establishment was sympathetic, but declared his proposals too risky and unrealistic. Ethical Prophets have insights to problems that no-one else can see. They can persuade the prevailing wisdom to change tack through their charisma and the authenticity of their belief. Newman was relentless and with an evangelical approach to the medical authorities. A breakthrough came when he converted an East Coast doyen of Paediatrics. Howard Pearson was an ideal convert, as he was one of the most distinguished Paediatricians of his time on the east coast of the USA. He was Professor and Chairman of the Department of Paediatrics at Yale University Medical School. He had been President of the American Academy of Paediatrics. He was the recipient of many honours and awards. He was on the editorial board of leading Paediatric journals and was author of textbooks and numerous articles. This patriarch of Paediatrics not only relented, but then became an enthusiastic supporter of the camps. He became the founding medical director of the Hole in the Wall Gang Camp and served from 1988 until 2002 (Pearson and Shefsky, 2015).

Notes

1 The photograph of five boys outside Lords before the 132-second annual cricket match between Eton and Harrow was taken by Jimmy Sime in 1937. Two boys on the left of the photo aged fourteen and fifteen wore top hats, tail coats, silk waistcoats and carried canes with an apparently arrogant stance of indifference towards three working-class boys on the right. The latter seem amused by the public school boys' pose. It is a superb photo that seems to epitomise the class divide in pre-war Britain. It has been variously described as 'the defining image of class division'; 'The Two Nations'; 'a symbol of arrogant privilege' and 'Toffs and Toughs'. Old photos carry the poignancy of the future disclosed. Every picture tells a story, but it was remarkably untrue. The taller boy of the pair on the right died a year later of diphtheria in India. The smaller 'Toff' became mentally unstable in the 1970s and in 1984 died in an asylum. The three 'Toughs' became prosperous, well-adjusted, contented men and were alive and well in 2010 (*Ian Jack, The Guardian, 2010*).

2 The Paul Newman quotations are taken from an interview with Matt Cook, Camp Director, Hole in the Wall Gang Camp (2008).

9   Genealogy of the camp embrace

Conditions of emergence

American Summer camps emerged in the nineteenth century in response to concern about modern youths' loss of the Frontier Spirit.
The camps adopted a 'back to nature' ideology. The first camps were
designed to toughen elite American manhood, but their remit in the
twentieth century became more democratic. Some camps developed a
therapeutic reputation after World War II, culminating in the development of Serious Fun camps. The American camp experience has been
suggested as a ritual process of change, but not in a way that utilises
van Gennep's concepts from Anthropology. The concept of liminality
resolves many of the debates around the importance of the Edenic trope.
Serious Fun camps utilise creative mimesis play but other camps depend
on mimesis imitation to reproduce preconceptions of an ideal. Masters
of Ceremonies are essential to guide the pharmakon of camp, as it can
be toxic as well as therapeutic.

> The genealogical method identifies two special concerns. One is the con-
> ceptualization of this emergence as a difference through the joining of two
> separate threads, while the other is to put emphasis on the conditions under
> which this linking has occurred.
>
> *Arpad Szakolczai*: Reflexive Historical Sociology

Serious Fun camps did not appear out of the blue. They were an adaptation of the American summer camp. A genealogical understanding needs
to trace the pedigree of Serious Fun camps from the initial emergence
of summer camps in the nineteenth century to the advent of specialised
camps for seriously ill children over 100 years later. The genealogy of
American summer camps emerged in conditions of rapid industrialisation
in the Northeastern United States associated with an increase in migrants
from Europe. There was a perceived threat to the American way of life
and concern about loss of the Frontier Spirit in American youths. Camp
ethos emerged from a belief that challenging experiences in the great
outdoors could reignite the pioneer spirit in young men distracted by the
machine age.

The first summer camps

The first summer camps in New England were Protestant islands of American virility. Health, rejuvenation and pioneer nostalgia connected campers to a romantic American tradition. Antimodern anxieties were translated into outdoor activity, health exercises and character development under the guidance of men as mentors, role models and counselors – effectively 'Masters of Ceremonies'. Rural recreation was promoted as a desirable antidote to the deleterious effects of city life. American summer camps were a solution to the effete city lives of the elite. In the eyes of the summer camp pioneers, Protestant youths had become pressurised and over regimented. They needed physical and spiritual restoration through a return to nature. The fashionable tour of Europe was being substituted by something more hardy and challenging. Extended, protected childhoods and antimodern anxiety propelled the camp ethos to a way of maintaining the superiority of the Puritan ideal (McNamara, 2009).

The rise of American summer camps

Leslie Paris (2008) traces the late nineteenth-century rise of American summer camps from their beginnings in the state of New York. Camps were initially confined to cadres of elite Protestant boys, who were thought to have lost the frontier spirit of the founding fathers. The camping ideal grew with each decade driven by notions of rural health benefits linked with opportunities to impart goals of good citizenship and social assimilation. In practice, the camps were socially segregated spaces until well into the twentieth century. Religion, gender and race served to separate children of different religions and ethnic groups so that family traditions remained sacrosanct, whilst the children became aware of common cultural aspirations. Camps were both sleep away and day camps. They served 'an American solution to the question of children's socialisation in modernity' (Paris, 2008:11). There were still less than 100 camps at the turn of the century in 1900, but rapid expansion led to the existence of over 1,000 camps by 1918 at the end of World War I (Smith, 2006). At the turn of the next century in 2001, over ten million American children experienced the pleasures of summer camp (Van Slyck, 2006).

Back-to-nature ideology

The essence of the camp experience was established in the nineteenth century. It entailed living away from home whilst participating in planned activities, evening camp fires and exposure to the natural world under the guidance of counselors. Different camps shared a desire to impart social values that had a common patriotic American orientation, but at the same time reflected a family's religious, educational and social values. The camps offered children opportunities for self-expression and communal living that may not have been available to them at home. Smith (2006) examined the different arguments about the benefits of camp through the twentieth century. From the beginning, those involved with the camping movement were very aware that these childhood holidays could be enduring transformative experiences. The belief was that the important circumstance was the back to nature ideal. This was an Edenic trope with survival challenges summarised by Kenneth Webb as an invitation to take the 'Great Leap Backward' (Smith, 2006:90). The values of exposure to nature were intuitive with the logic that the camp was a better world than urban existence. When some camps introduced entertainment facilities such as the cinema, they were pilloried as a guiding principle of camp was to be in opposition to civilisation. Camps were soon purged of urban recreational activities.

Child psychology

G. Stanley Hall, a pioneer of child psychology, proposed a theory of childhood as a recapitulation of cultural progress. Stages of child development were reflected in maturation of different nations ranging from 'savages' to the uber civilised in the Western World. In other words, children had to go through a stage of 'savagery' or surviving in the wild in order to become civilised. Hall's book *Adolescence* published in 1904 was very influential and a great boost to the camping movement (Arnett, 2006). 'Childhood is a biological and developmental category' (Paris, 2008:14) that varies in different eras and places. Hall made an analogy with Ernst Haeckel's theory about embryonic development recapitulating evolution as already discussed in Chapter 7, but Hall's recapitulation was about cultural progress in the refining process of civilisation rather than the natural process of evolution. It was in tune with Lamarck's idea that acquired characteristics are passed on to the next generation. Darwin anticipated modern genetics just as Lamarck anticipated the centrality of mimesis in child development. For Hall, gender was another track of development with incomplete maturation of boys being especially risky. Hall's theory of development was 'essentially a male narrative of progress and civilisation' (Paris, 2008:29) and the camp was somehow an effective way of ensuring successful transition to manhood. Camp leaders in the early twentieth century drew satisfaction from a scientific gloss provided by Hall's theory of developmental child psychology that seemed to support the importance of a counter modern experience in the healthy socialisation of children: it confirmed the need for an antidote to city life. The back-to-nature ideal of camping endured a century of profound change. Nature was presumed to be the necessary catalyst for the effectiveness of the camp experience.

Camp agendas

The melting pot ideal towards a common American patriotism was initially unavailable as camps reflected religious, wealth, racial and educational divides. It was to some extent met by the gradual democratisation of the camp embrace in the first half of the twentieth century. Then camps expanded their constituency and sought not only to toughen the elite, but also to uplift the poor and heal the sick through deliberate socialisation of values. The remit of camps broadened into largely separate strands of private and organisational camps. Organisational camps with a cultural agenda such as the YMCA were largely religious. Many advocates regarded child-centred camps with nature-orientated programmes as the corrective to social pathologies of modern civilisation such as various forms of moral, spiritual and physical turpitude. Smith (2006) achieves a resolution to this twentieth century debate about the importance of the natural world in reforming children's beliefs and values. He suggested that the important aspect of camp was an intense experience of difference. This was a back-to-nature environment for city dwelling children. Camps helped define American childhood as a special space. 'Growth could be fertilized by intense experiences' (Smith, 2006:94), making camp an ideal environment to explore and test new values.

Social transformations

The value of camp was uncontested, but its transformative capacity remained a mystery. Arnold van Gennep published *Les Rites de Passage* in 1908. It was not translated into English until 1960. His discovery of liminality and its contemporary relevance (Thomassen, 2014) to the transformative capacity of camp had not informed the debate – due to its relative obscurity and a lack of an English translation. Leslie Paris (2008) in her book *Children's Nature, The Rise of the American Summer Camp* comes close to describing the American summer camp as a rite of passage, but makes no reference to van Gennep's detailed analysis of the necessary conditions and mechanisms that assist social transformations in tribal societies:

> At their best camps could feel like magical spaces, fundamentally unexplainable to outsiders, where pleasure and improvement were conjoined (Paris, 2008:4) ...Camp culture comprised a series of rites of passage, some more formal or explicit than others, designed to foster children's sense of participating in a transformative enterprise... These differences allowed camps to feel like miniature worlds apart from the everyday, worlds where life was lived fully and intensely.
>
> (ibid:98)

Leslie Paris recognised that camps could be an intense, fleeting and transformative experience away from the routine of school. As far as can be judged she takes the concept of a 'rite of passage' as a common description of change rather than a reference from Anthropology. Paris (2008) did not have the concept of liminality, which would have resolved the debate around the Edenic trope. Parents approved of country air and the maturational role of camps. Camps endorsed the idea that childhood should be a time apart separated from adult culture. The need for counselors was established from the beginning. Intense and challenging experiences supported by counselors were integral to the camp. It was 'the ideal space for clarifying values, testing them and deciding which ones were worth carrying back to the real world' (Smith, 2006:94).

The nineteenth-century founders of the camp in the New World, inspired by nostalgia for the frontier spirit, stumbled on ancient anthropological mechanisms of social transformation. Smith claims that the summer camp leaders understood in an inchoate way that it was the "contrast" between the child's everyday world and the camp world that enhanced the children's growth and development'. The founders of the American summer camp reproduced by serendipity the important conditions for rites of passage. The back-to-nature ideal provided *separation* from their everyday world; intense challenging experiences guided by counselors promoted social *transformation*, and camping ideals imagined the children's *re-integration* back into their urban lives.

Camp as a therapeutic milieu

After World War II, some camps developed a therapeutic reputation. The abiding premise of the camping movement from its origins in the nineteenth century was a belief that the machine age was enfeebling American manhood. The camp associations had fortuitously assembled a transformative process with a rite of passage structure based on nostalgia for the frontier spirit, which could be recaptured in a back-to-nature format. The Austrian child psychologist Fritz Redl, trained by Anna Freud, emigrated to the USA aged thirty-four in 1936. After the war, he was Clinical Director at the University of Michigan Fresh Air Camp for several summers. He introduced a cautionary note into romantic notions about the camp experience (Smith, 2006). The environment of camp could have a downside as well as beneficial effects. Redl regarded the back-to-nature ideology as a hodgepodge of Indian lore. Perhaps his most important insight was that the camp had the nature of a pharmakon, so that it could be toxic as well as therapeutic. Home sickness was a problem for a few, and a small minority loathed their time in camp. For Riedl, the idea that nature was a healer could be inverted as the natural world could also be alien and threatening to campers. Nonetheless most children were exhilarated by camp experiences and cherished their memories of outdoor excitement and camaraderie. Redl understood that the therapeutic effect of camp was not the experience of nature *per se*, but in the nature of the experience, which was a tripartite process of separation, transition and re-integration: the experience of a rite of passage.

The Hole in the Wall Gang Camp

The Hole in the Wall Gang Camp was the first purpose built holiday facility for seriously ill children. Sick children had been previously accepted in some camps, but nobody had dared harbour a camp full of one of the most feared childhood illnesses prior to 1988. The camp has a wonderful location in Ashford, Connecticut, and the facilities there are like most other camps.

Newman's innovations were few but important. The key was a medical service called the Infirmary in OK corral that had excellent facilities and highly qualified medical staff available around the clock. It was unobtrusive but reassured parents and discreetly provided care and treatment as necessary. The stature and reputation of Dr Howard Pearson as the founding medical director was sufficient to gain the confidence of referring Paediatricians. Newman's second innovation was to increase the number of counselors, so that the child/counselor ratio was often one to one. That was based on the simple idea that seriously ill children needed more care, but it also ensured that a unique role model relationship could develop between campers and counselors even in the short duration of camp. The Hole in the Wall Gang Camp name comes from Newman's favourite film *Butch Cassidy and the Sundance Kid*. Newman wanted the camp to be like 'The Hole in the Wall Pass' in Wyoming, which served as a refuge and hideout for outlaws in the movie. He envisaged a location that could likewise be a refuge and hideout where seriously ill children could 'raise a little hell' (Pearson and Shefsky, 2016).

Serious Fun camps expanded through the USA and the concept of camp catering for seriously ill children was taken up by other organisations. By the time Newman's friends in Hollywood went fund raising for a purpose-built camp in California, they found that there were already four camps there serving children with life-threatening conditions in Paediatric Haematology and Oncology. They looked for new challenges and as only Hollywood can they dreamed up a wonderful camp called the Painted Turtle.

The Painted Turtle

The Painted Turtle camp in California opened in 2004 and was built for purpose. It is in a dry mountain area and caters for diverse medical disorders unlike the Hole in the Wall, which mainly caters for children with cancer and leukaemia. In both camps, the basic elements of a rite of passage described by vanGennep and Turner can be easily recognised.

At first glance, it may be difficult to see what the Painted Turtle and the magnificent Getty Museum in Los Angeles have in common. The Painted Turtle is in a dry mountain area about seventy miles northeast of Los Angeles. The Getty lords it over Hollywood and beyond. The museum houses cultural treasures from all over the world, whereas the important residents in the Painted Turtle are children with serious chronic illnesses. The Getty stands as a magnificent citadel overlooking Los Angeles like the Parthenon on the Acropolis; the Painted Turtle blends into the California countryside like an ancient African Village. Despite this contrast, they were both designed by Richard Meier and are at the same time magnificent statements of a well-considered dynamic between function and form. The museum stands in the foothills of the Santa Monica Mountains and is designed to be seen. The Painted Turtle is near Lake Hughes, but needs a double take by passers-by to recognise the camping community. The Painted Turtle's link with the Getty Museum hints at a search for excellence: seeking the best available architect to plan a further development in Serious Fun camps for sick children. In 1998, the Association of the Hole in the Wall Gang Camps did a needs assessment of the camping experiences of children with medically complex diseases in California. Serious illnesses not served were renal failure, liver transplantation, muscular dystrophy, Crohn's disease, ulcerative colitis, diabetes mellitus, congenital heart disease, skeletal dysplasia and thalassaemia; the Painted Turtle planned a camping experience for children with these complex conditions. Perhaps chronic renal failure was the most difficult condition to replicate a safe camping experience from a paediatric perspective. The Painted Turtle was designed from scratch, so they built medical systems into the buildings. Peritoneal dialysis reservoirs were plumbed into the cabins. This enabled children to stay in bed and be full-time campers during dialysis. The process worked unheard and unseen and the filtration water went directly to sewage. At full stretch the renal camp caters for twenty-five children on haemodialysis and another twenty-five on peritoneal dialysis as outlined by the medical director:

> The idea of building the systems into the buildings was an important part of this camp's creation. During that session, we have an entire team that just does haemodialysis. The haemodialysis unit from St Joseph's of Orange, their entire team comes up here. We have the Department of Health and Human Services that has to review all the lab tests on the water that we use prior to haemodialysis. They have to look at all of the certifications of the people that are going to be running the haemodialysis. We have an entire team that does peritoneal dialysis because it's all done overnight. We have a team that stays up all night long and is able to troubleshoot the machines as the alarms go off and that type of thing. So we have a team that's up all night, we have got a team that is just doing haemodialysis, and then we have an entire team that gives out the medication; because these children are on up to fifteen and twenty medications three or four times a day. It's an exhausting, amazing web of medical providers trying not to be seen. The kids have a blast.

The counselors remain camper focussed. These are '*children* with kidney disease and not nephrology *patients*'. The Painted Turtle has enabled children with very difficult medical conditions such as renal failure and muscular dystrophy to have the kind of camping experience favoured by Serious Fun camps. The renal failure camp is a triumph for the planners and technical support teams. The muscular dystrophy camp is a tribute to the dedication of young counselors. The children with muscular dystrophy pose great practical difficulties, and yet for many of the counselors, it is their most fulfilling camp:

> Most fulfilling is muscular dystrophy because like J said, its seeing what they are going through, and being able to appreciate just taking a step in the morning.

One of the coolest things was for Muscular Dystrophy, was these kids – how vulnerable – they have to have everything done for them; and so to come to a camp where 20–30 year old people who are not trained in that, to change them. Like I could not imagine having someone else do those types of things for me. I think it's also something that they are so giving. It's an experience where they give to us as well. How are you going to lift a 300lb kid, if you are going to wipe someone's butt, how are you going to do that?

If the muscular dystrophy was the most fulfilling camp, the diabetic camp posed intrusive problems for the counselors:

I suppose the only week that really sticks out for me besides MDA (muscular dystrophy association) would be diabetes week. It's just because diabetes week is really hard compared to other weeks because they have to do checks every so often. It does not feel like normal camp.

Another counselor identified the problem as a clash between medical and social responsibilities:

The medical stuff comes into the cabins. That I think is what makes it the hardest. The doctors and the nurses are coming up and you are doing carb counts and you are doing that. I think it's hard because it's a lot harder to keep that focus that it's camp, because you are watching them prick their fingers and putting blood into a machine throughout the day; the different stations and worrying about that; it makes you realise what they are going through. It makes it a little harder to make sure that you are focusing on the camp portion while keeping them healthy. We have to see if they go low in between those checks…

In the diabetic camp, the medical aspect should in theory be confined to the Well Shell, but it was a pervasive presence in the cabin:

Even the fact you know for that week it's kind of a thing where for us it's that social aspect – the medicine is always in the well shell. When in that first week we had someone with diabetes, maybe because it was those steroids she was on, she developed it, but to have that stuff in cabin all the time, you know I mean like, it just puts you on a different awareness. I think it just shifts your thought processes and medical comes first.

The rite of separation was incomplete as the hospital world intruded on the camp experience for the children with diabetes and their counselors. It is interesting that most holiday camps for children with diabetes have an educational emphasis (McAuliffe-Fogarty et al., 2007), as if the only way to cope with the condition is to master it.

The Painted Turtle may seem a strange name for a camp, but makes sense when explained by a senior member of staff:

> When the planners were looking for property in California the first place they looked was on painted horse road. The amalgam came because the word turtle had been very important in our founder's family. The Painted Turtle is an actual animal that by happy coincidence has been a brilliant representation of the camp… the turtle is such a non-threatening creature but warm and wise and fun and people don't get tired of it. I think it has been a great representation of the Painted Turtle. There are stories about it, there is history, there is lore in different cultures, and the turtle is always one of those foundation animals that people trust and feel comfortable with.

The recognition factor of a Painted Turtle was important for spreading the word about the camp. The camping experience was easily symbolised as a parting gift of a painted turtle pillow at the end of the camp. This portable symbol like the hope represented by a miraculous medal or a scapular in a traditional Catholic culture serves as a reminder of better times for children when they have to face further challenging experiences in hospitals.

Serious Fun camps

The tripartite ritual experiences of separation, liminality and re-integration integral to the American Camping Experience can be seen in Serious Fun camps with different degrees of emphasis. The Painted Turtle in California, the Hole in the Wall Gang Camp in Connecticut and Barretstown in Ireland are almost mirror images of one another in that they adhere to the principles of complete separation from home and hospital, a liminal phase distinguished by transformative experiences in a spirit of communitas, and a process of re-integration as the children are encouraged to incorporate their camping experiences on return to their everyday world. The experience may be sub-optimal when these traditional principals cannot be sustained. Some camps have outreach programmes that attempt to recapture the camp experience in hospitals.

Outreach

A number of camps have attempted an outreach service to try and bring the experience into hospitals. This might seem an impossible task if credence is given to the importance of rites of separation, transformation and re-integration. The Connecticut camp continues to visit hospitals, but the style of interaction has changed to an individual bedside level that inevitably lacks the distinctive communitas of camps. The Painted Turtle has had the most success. The symbol excites inpatients: 'the Painted Turtle, the Painted Turtle!'

A senior member of staff who developed the outreach programme for the Painted Turtle emphasises the communal aspect by trying to get the children to play together:

These two kids ran into the playroom and they had done it before and said let me set up the lake. So they helped me set up the lake and the fishing because they knew. They had been there before. It was very much like camp. Like we are on day three and the campers suddenly know how to set the table themselves. They know how to set the dishes. They know how to do cabin clean up. So that's been really nice. We were having an effect that we were hitting them more than one time and they were remembering us. They ask us are we coming back tomorrow. 'Oh you will come back tomorrow'.

The small team from the Painted Turtle do not forget the hospital staff:

I always try to leave something at the hospital like flowers for all the nurses with all their names on, tissue paper flowers, which were really easy but you would have thought that we had given them gold. The next time we came back it was 'Hi Painted Turtle, the Painted Turtle is back'. They remembered.

All children's hospitals have or should have play therapists, because somebody needs to mediate the challenges of upsetting hospital experiences. A lot of emphasis is placed on ensuring that procedures are not intimidating or painful. It can be more difficult to alleviate the social isolation of some hospital experiences. The Painted Turtle outreach programmes are aware that their expertise, based on camp know-how, can neutralise the children's social estrangement from the hospital world:

Most children in hospital are self-absorbed, and it is the social aspect of camp that can transform the hospital for a while. They are kind of involved in their own world. So that social addition, and to me that aspect is so important to us and to meet is good for this program; because I feel that is a real need in a hospital is to have that social addition time.

The Painted Turtle programme tries to bring their rites of passage into hospital. The separation has already happened through hospital admission, and then there can be an undertow of liminal dread as the children detach from their home and family. The outreach programme tries to introduce the communitas of camp:

So we get them to interact with each other that slowly starts to build just like it does at camp. It's on a much smaller level but it's still happening. By the end of the two hours that we are with them, we had gathered around camp fire. We were making rainstorms to put out the camp fire and singing the songs about where we all come from and how nice it was to share and meet friends and be together for the day. You could see how, on the kid's faces, that they really felt something. They felt the connection somehow really was to meet friends, to meet us; they were smiling for the first time, maybe it was a distraction for two hours where we transported them to a different place where we were fishing and I had the camp music on. It's very important to have that on in the background.

It does seem that the benefit of the programme requires previous experience of the camp. This is not so much of a problem in the USA, where the feeling of the camp spirit is part of their culture:

> I really think that the kids get it. We talk about – no matter where you are – camp is always in your heart and as a human being you can take it with you; More than anything it's the whole package: the feel we bring them, the music, the energy, the games, the positivity. I think we just bowl them over with camp spirit. I think what camp does best, what makes camp so powerful is that we create this community that is a total society. We take the best of the world and bring it here and don't let anything upset it. We just don't.

Parents deeply appreciate the visit. They themselves are often bored out of their mind with the mundane routine of hospital visiting. They recognise the restoration of their child's spirit:

> They are sick of hospital for days and days and days… the father that was there; he just kept saying to us 'God bless you for doing this, thank you for being here and bringing this to my family'. You could see that he was very moved by what we were doing.

The Painted Turtle outreach team seems to have achieved the impossible by at least partially reproducing the experience of the camp in hospitals. The crucial step seems to have been an ability to recreate the spirit of communitas, which can energise the children's flagging spirit.

The idea of bringing the camping experience back into hospital has led to many practical difficulties. The repetition of a rite of passage tripartite structure is an almost insurmountable obstacle within a hospital. The nearest reproduction of camp has been achieved by the Painted Turtle outreach programme. They have the advantage of an instantly recognisable symbol that communicates the spirit of camp, which facilitates the establishment of a temporary environment of liminality and communitas. The outreach staff of the Painted Turtle endeavour to recreate a communal rather than an individual engagement with inpatients. These factors may be why the Painted Turtle has had the most success with an outreach programme.

The spirit of the camp embrace

Serious Fun camps can be conceived as short-term total institutions that inspire reinvigoration of children who have had life-challenging experiences because of their chronic severe illnesses. The circumstances of camp resemble a rite of passage, but the ritual process acquires its formative force from the spirit of camp mimed and guided by Counselors and Caras as Masters of Ceremonies. The guiding force of change in the children's spirit is mimetic and largely sub-conscious. The question arises as to what is distinctive about Serious Fun camps from other transformative camps loosely labelled as boot camps. The literary theorist Mihai Spariosu (1997) drew a distinction between mimesis imitation and mimesis play that echoes Merlin Donald's evolution of communication through increasing sophistication of the mimetic process. Mimetic commu-nication starts as a reflex (tongue protrusion in the newborn), followed by repetition (smiling, babbling) to creative symbols (pointing, knowing winks, questioning eyebrows) that provide a foundation for speech. Mimesis imitation (repetition) and mimesis play (creativity) may help draw a distinction between the spirits of different camp styles. Camps that have a preconceived image of outcomes such as weight loss targets in fitness camps, the attributes of a marine or learning goals in educational camps all aim at repetition of an ideal. On the other hand, camps that nourish creativity have more personal and healing goals that respond to individual needs. Serious Fun camps do not have any precon-ceived images for their camping alumni other than a salutogenic orientation to the world. In contrast, the Imus Ranch exemplified a camp that had an aim of repetition of an ideal conceived as the 'Great American Cowboy'.

The Imus Ranch

The Imus Ranch (1999–2014) was a camp based in New Mexico that merits comment as it had a distinctive approach based on the beliefs of its founders – Don and Deirdre Imus. The Imus ranch sought to provide a special experi-ence of the 'Great American Cowboy' for sick children and their siblings. The ranch had tenuous connections with Serious Fun camps as the idea of a ranch experience came to Imus (a radio talk show celebrity) during research for an interview with Paul Newman.

The ranch is fifty miles southeast of Santa Fe on 4,000 acres. It was featured in *Architectural Digest*, an international magazine of interior design (Collins, 2001). The Imus Ranch opened in 1999 and closed in 2014. The ranch ac-cepted ten children per week during the summer, but was a working cattle ranch throughout the year. The Imus family were volunteers at the ranch and Don Imus broadcasted his radio programme from there. It was not a Serious Fun camp as children had to do chores, care for horses and feed the animals. The children experienced working on the ranch (Lerner, 2010). The Imus Ranch could be exhausting as it operated from sunrise to sunset. Deirdre and Don Imus made it clear that their aim was to instil the values of hard work. 'We're straight shooters with these kids', says Deirdre: 'We lay down the rules the first day here: "This isn't Camp Happy Face"' (Keel, 2005).

There were hard learned lessons during a week at the ranch. Only two of ten children won prizes – one for the best overall time in rodeo, and one for displaying the best attitude during his or her stay. 'In life, everyone isn't always a winner', Mr Imus told his new ranch hands (Lerner, 2010). Ranch policy forbids mention of illness. Everyone stays in the big house like one family. 'Almost to a kid it's the experience of their life', says Imus. The accommodation is luxurious with no 'crummy cabins' unlike most camps.

Two child life specialists were in continuous attendance together with a medical presence. In 2004, Dr Howard Pearson, the first medical director of the Hole in the Wall Gang Camp in Connecticut, worked there for a short period as a paid physician in charge of medical care. A strange altercation arose between Dr Pearson and Don Imus during the camp because of a call to see a child who complained of pain. The infirmary was less than a five-minute walk and en route Dr Pearson declined a lift from Deirdre Imus. Don Imus subsequently screamed at Pearson for ten minutes in front of several children and adults. He repeatedly described Howard Pearson on his radio programme as 'an arrogant fucking doctor who doesn't mind letting a child suffer' (Wikipedia, 2017). Pearson sued Imus for slander and civic assault in July 2006.

The ranch's list of contributors was not public information although funded through public donations and corporations. In addition to donations, the ranch is run on profits from an annual radio fund raising, the sale of Imus ranch foods and non-toxic home agents. The cost per child works out at $27,000 or roughly ten times the cost to send a child to the Hole in the Wall Gang Camp in Connecticut.

The ranch had some parallels with Serious Fun camps but was seriously problematic in several respects. Don and Deirdre Imus had a hands-on role in managing the ranch experience, and were effectively Masters of Ceremonies. There was complete separation from the outside world and cell phones were forbidden. The children were separated from their former life, but the ranch mixed domestic life of the family with the ritual space of a rite of passage. The ritual activities of transformation in Serious Fun camps were replaced by routine chores that belong to the everyday world. The Imus ranch fits the model of a tripartite experience, but the liminal experience was different: rather than suspension of normal rules and everyday reality facilitating communitas and Agape, the experience of Imus was as a kind of indoctrination with values of the 'Great American Cowboy'. Everyone is a winner in Serious Fun camps, but only two of ten children were winners in the Imus Ranch. The mode of interaction was competitive rather than cooperative. A compulsory vegetarian diet determined by the beliefs of Deirdre Imus may not have suited all children. In this confused and confusing situation neither separation from the everyday nor communitas, nor social transformation are possible. The experience was predetermined by the ethic of the 'Great American Cowboy'. The formative influence in the Ranch was unregulated mimesis-imitation rather than the inspirational spontaneity of mimesis-play in Serious Fun camps. The Imus Ranch for Sick Children closed in 2014, whilst Serious Fun International has grown from strength to strength.

10 Serious Fun International

Word spread like wildfire that the Hole in the Wall Gang Camp had beneficial effects on children with cancer and leukaemia. Sick children were sent from Ireland and elsewhere so that Newman recognised a need for a camp in Europe. The Irish camp in Barretstown castle opened in 1994. The excitement and enthusiasms of American Camps did not transfer easily to Europe, but was facilitated by the 'Therapeutic Recreation' framework that guided staff members through the camp sessions. There are now nine Serious Fun camps in the United States, five in Europe, eight in Africa, one each in Haiti, Israel, India, Cambodia, Vietnam and Japan. The Serious Fun network has become truly international and a Global Partnership Program links with the poorest countries ensuring that the benefits of Serious Fun camps are not confined to affluent countries. All camps have a Rite of Passage structure that optimises beneficial social change.

> Barretstown opened in 1994 and catered for 128 children that geared up to 350 children in 1995. Barretstown relied on five American counselors in the first year, which helped initiate the first European counselors into the spirit and guided spontaneity of summer camp. The English, German, French and Irish needed the American model to get them going.
>
> *The Baxter Foundation Report 1996*

This chapter will outline how Paul Newman's vision was exported first to Ireland and then to the rest of the world. The know-how of the American camp lifestyle as a modern tradition since the late nineteenth century is taken for granted in the USA. In contrast, European children are less familiar with the camp. However, it should be borne in mind that Baden Powell founded the Boy Scouts in 1908; the Girl Guides followed in 1910, with several million members in the UK, France, Germany, Belgium, Scandinavia, etc. As well, there have been numerous camp movements throughout Europe, in the 1920s to 1940s especially, which are very similar to the American camp movement in their explicitly ideological purpose and their 'back to nature' ethos. The significant difference between the European and the American camp movements is that, generally, the European camp movements became disreputable due to their association with Fascism and Communism, whereas American camp ideology associated with a masculine Christianity retained an essentially benign culture of an optimistic world. Even the values of the 'Great American Cowboy' promulgated in the Imus Ranch are not questioned apart from Don Imus' style of implementation, which was problematic for the needs of seriously ill children.

The experience and perspective of European Serious Fun campers can still contribute to the unique nature of sick children's experience of camp and highlight aspects that American children take for granted. In Barretstown, the children's spatial, temporal and psychological separation from their home in many parts of Europe is striking. Instantaneous recognition of common treatment protocols alleviates the shock of new experiences and triggers liminal feelings of fellowship amongst campers from different countries. The medical conventions that have ruled their lives are suddenly relaxed and made objects of fun. There are no apparent titles or visible rank amongst the staff; all social exchanges are in first names only. The whole experience bears an uncanny resemblance to the classic descriptions of rites of passage in *The Rites of Passage* by Arnold van Gennep (1960) and *The Ritual Process* by Victor Turner (1969).

Barretstown, the first European camp

After the Hole in the Wall Gang Camp opened in 1988, the word spread like wildfire that the experience had beneficial effects on children with cancer and leukaemia. By the following year, the first child from Ireland had been sent to the camp in Connecticut by Cancer Radiotherapist Dr Ian Fraser:

> So I picked a young lad who was a very resilient young lad, who had gone back to his uncle's farm at the weekend. He worked on the farm and came up here for radiation therapy, and a big lad, a quiet lad but resilient. I felt that if it is not right, if the thing is not kosher, this kid would be OK. So the parents were two primary school teachers. And I went out to the airport to send this kid off and he went off to America. He had ten days in the camp and he had a couple of days in New York and he came back. I was at the airport when he came back and I watched him go out and I watched him come back and he was a different child. And the mother said 'this isn't my child. This child has confidence. This child …there is something about him… a sense of independence which he did not have before.'

Other children followed to the extent that Paul Newman realised that there needed to be a camp in Europe. The initial plan was to locate the camp in the UK or France, but Ian Fraser flew to the States and contacted Newman's lawyer Carroll W. Brewster. He persuaded him to visit Ireland:

> We got the message that Brewster was coming to Ireland. He said look, you guys have to find us a castle. In America its cowboys and Indians, in

Europe it's got to be a castle. I went to my brother, who is a business man and my brother went to the Office of Public Works, who said we have this place down the country Barretstown.

Newman came to Ireland and when he saw Barretstown he said, 'when I first saw Barretstown Castle I knew this was where I wanted the first European camp to be'. Ireland unlike America is full of doubting Thomases:

> The Office of Public Works thought no more have I got Newman than I have the man in the moon. But when Newman walked around the corner of the castle, he has a very characteristic profile; the boys were sitting on the grass chatting away about all sorts of stuff. And the boys looked over at Newman and said, 'Jesus this is a runner, this is going'. We went in and had lunch and we were so nervous about this. I was terrified, I couldn't swallow. Because I thought this is on the cusp. And we had a good lunch. We had a great chat with Newman. On the way out he spotted a can of Budweiser. He turned around to me and said, 'do you guys drink Budweiser'. We said we drink everything, we drink loads of Budweiser. He said, 'I'll get you some money'. He went back to America, rang a guy called Micky Rourke, and Rourke was the second in command of Anheuser–Busch. And he explained the situation that this pair had got a castle in Ireland backed by the Irish government and could Anheuser–Busch give us some money. So Rourke said I'll give you $800,000. So that was the start.

In 1994, as reported in the New York Times, Paul Newman signed a lease on Barretstown Castle with Albert Reynolds, the Prime Minister of Ireland:

> Under the terms of the 99-year lease, the Irish Government will collect one Irish pound, or about $1.50, each year from the Barretstown Castle Gang Camp, which will occupy the 500-acre premises, where sheep and cattle roam.

Caras and Anam Caras

Barretstown had of necessity a strong American influence as there was no tradition of camp in Ireland. In some ways, the exuberant optimism of the USA had to be toned down a little:

> It is an American institution, like we didn't grow up with it. They grew up with it. They had to be here at the beginning…but Barretstown needed to move towards a more European feel… You tone it down like. One of the things we would always say especially for our family camps and particularly our bereavement camps, when it's their first camp…you are not out in front of the castle like lunatics jumping up and down…

because they are Irish people. They don't want to see that...they will just keep driving and drive back out the gates again. Just be a little bit more reserved until they get used to it. You can then get them up dancing and doing skits and stuff like that. You have to ease them into it a little bit slower than you'd do over in America. (Clinical Director, *The Med Shed Barretstown*).

American Counselors and their expertise were absorbed into the Irish scene and renamed as Caras. A *Cara* is the Gaelic for friend and their relationship with campers can be better described as an *Anam Cara* that translates as a soul mate and a mentor. The first Hole in the Wall Gang Camp in Connecticut was designed to cater for children with cancer or leukaemia, and these were the commonest disorders seen in Barretstown. These illnesses affect social class indiscriminately. The one exception was a week that catered for children who had AIDS and tended to come from less fortunate socio-economic circumstances. Happily that condition has almost disappeared from children due to effective treatment during pregnancy. All children in camp still have or have recovered from a life-threatening illness. Their experiences of ill health are similar because they will have been treated by similar protocols despite their diverse backgrounds from all over Europe. Their morbidity is largely a consequence of treatment by chemotherapy, radiotherapy and surgery, rather than the underlying illness.

Access to the holiday camp is dependent on hospital referral. Barretstown has a well-defined philosophy of care. The principle of non-discrimination informs the work ethic and all programmes are provided free of charge. Funding is dependent on the support and generosity of individuals, corporations and foundations. When Barretstown opened in 1994, it catered for 128 children and since then has gradually expanded catering for over 1,400 children and families in the year 2000, over 1,500 in 2005 and 2,700 by 2015. The facility can cater for over 100 children with serious illnesses and over 100 staff and volunteers at any one session.

A 1999 outline of a plan for a perfect day in Barretstown is a summary that all American counselors would recognise, because even five years after the camp opened in Ireland, the zeitgeist of Barretstown retained the spirit of the original American style that is still there today. The record of a perfect summer's day in 1999 was left in the castle's 'Harry Potter drawer'. It reveals an action packed programme with special times for reflection.

A perfect day

7.30am – 8.30am EARLY BIRDS: Challenge by choice is a fundamental principle of Barretstown. Early birds is all about choice. Children get to choose a special activity before breakfast.

8.30am – 9.00am: RISE AND SHINE: Showers, shampoo, socks and shoes and off to breakfast with a song.

9.00am – 10.00am BREAKFAST: Cornflakes for the campers, croissants and coffee for the Caras. Everyone charges their batteries for the day's activities, important announcements are made, where to meet, who lost a jumper, weather reports. Then the kids and the Caras help tidy away the breakfast dishes.

9.00am – 10.00am COTTAGE CLEAN UP: They find fun in every job that must be done.

10.30am ACTIVITY ASSEMBLY: Cottage groups are gender specific, the activity groups consist of boys and girls of a similar age that adds peer socialisation to all activities.

10.30am – 1.00pm ACTIVITIES: Canoeing, creative writing, taking pictures, horse riding, high ropes. Will they succeed? Yes.

1.00pm – 2.00pm LUNCH: It's a noisy boisterous time with singing, skits and silliness; as well as lunch.

2.00pm – 3.30pm REST TIME: Camp days are packed to the rafters with activity and it's important to give the campers and the Caras a bit of a rest. This is a chance for the campers to relax in their cottages, have a nap, do a jigsaw puzzle, write postcards, Peace and quiet.

3.30pm – 4.15pm CRAZY AND LAZY: This is when the Caras creativity flourishes – a time for the campers to try something weird and wonderful – outside the structured activity schedule. Juggling, dressing up in outlandish costumes.

4.15pm – 6.00pm SPECIAL PROJECT: This is a time for campers to spend time on a project they really enjoy and an opportunity to bring home a lasting memory of Barretstown.

6.00pm – 7.00pm DINNER: The amiable nurses stroll around doling out the meds.

EVENING PROGRAM: The evening program is an all camp activity that usually occurs in the theatre: various schemes for each cottage to display their talents to the rest of the camping community.

COTTAGE CHATS: Reflection is an important aspect of therapeutic recreation and the cottage chats provide an excellent opportunity for reflecting on the successes of the day and to discuss any other issues that may arise in an emotionally safe environment. The Caras encourage discussion without intruding.

LIGHTS OUT: Time varies – age dependent.

The 'perfect day' is a model for camp activities that would easily be recognised today in America or anywhere else in the world that have established Serious Fun camps. Thirty years after the original Hole in the Wall Gang Camp opened in 1988, different Serious Fun camps in America and the rest of the world have their own local variations, but the outline of the 'perfect day' remains a blueprint for all camps. Serious Fun camps are total institutions, but with important distinctions from Goffman's description (Goffman, 1997) that the duration is brief and there is no humiliation. The camp embrace is affectionate, caring and inspiring. It has an agenda of personal development through challenging achievements, but the challenges are by choice and tailored to suit individual abilities of sick children so that unknown to the child success is a guaranteed outcome. Activities range from the excitement of high ropes to creativity in arts and crafts, but whatever their choice the Caras and activity leaders carefully guide the children through the challenges.

The establishment of Serious Fun camps in the USA was relatively easy as they were a continuation of a long tradition, but this was not true when Paul Newman decided to bring Serious Fun camps to Europe. Counselors are the heart and soul of the American camp experience and their expertise easily transferred to the special needs of the Hole in the Wall Gang Camp in Connecticut. The situation in Ireland was different when the first European camp opened six years later in Barretstown. In Ireland, there was no reservoir of counselors that could be easily trained up for the smooth running of camp for seriously ill children. The enthusiastic camping culture would be difficult to replicate in Ireland. The immediate remedy was to import American counselors to kick start the camping lifestyle. American camp culture had to be imported and translated into a more reserved European style.

American counselors needed an *aide memoire* for their European counterparts who would be recruited every year and trained into the ethos of the American summer camp. One of the first American counselors in Barretstown had trained in Therapeutic Recreation and saw the potential of that approach to guide Europeans about the camp. Therapeutic Recreation proved to be an excellent cultural bridge and has proved very helpful for European countries unfamiliar with American camp culture. It gives Caras an enthusiastic attitude towards children that effectively simplifies camping activities into a number of stages. Barretstown needed Therapeutic Recreation as it catered for campers from all over Europe, none of whom had any familiarity with the camping lifestyle. Therapeutic Recreation is now held in great esteem by European camps as it is given credit for being the source of a change in the children's quality of life (Bekesi et al., 2011).

Therapeutic Recreation

Barretstown gradually became distinct from its sister camps in the USA through its emphasis on Therapeutic Recreation. Bator Tabor camp in Hungary and Over the Wall in the UK have followed suit. Therapeutic Recreation deliberately formulates social action and efficacy into a memorable sequence. The campers are completely unaware that a special sequence guides their interaction with Caras. The philosophy of Therapeutic Recreation (Peterson and Stumbo, 2000) underpins these activities following a model of *Challenge, Success, Reflection,* and *Discovery*. The children choose a challenge based on their abilities. The challenges are structured to ensure success. The children reflect on their experience at the end of the day and discover their previously compromised or unrecognised potential. There are fourteen core activities including canoeing, archery, horse riding, arts and crafts and creative writing. A staff member commented that the children's achievements surprise not only themselves, but also health professionals:

> Even the doctors are surprised at what the children can do here. Doctors find that they can do more things than they thought children could do when they are on leukaemia treatment, and along with everyone else their eyes are opened when they see the children whiz up the high ropes with a prosthetic femur.

Each activity offers a kind of a challenge, often confronting the campers with an unknown situation, which encourages them to step over their real or imagined limitations, and try themselves out in new situations. The completion of the challenges is always accompanied by success and recognition – this process is facilitated by the encouraging attitude and supportive attention of volunteer and professional staff. In the morning, the Caras present the challenge by agreeing with the children what they are going to do that day. The challenge outlined by a senior staff member in Barretstown is by choice:

> Each child is challenged to the limit of his or her ability within the group. In some subtle way, they make sure that they succeed. It happens because of the tremendous skill of the staff. It's easy enough to set challenges, and I suppose it's easy enough to make everybody succeed in their challenge. The subtle bit is to make them feel that they themselves have succeeded rather than being helped along. To some extent, they 'rediscover their childhood'… 'the discovery element comes right through the programme. What they are doing is different from what they thought they could do'. In this discovery, the children learn to 'redefine themselves'.
>
> Every activity is debriefed…you actually make time to reflect and establish a reality for the child about their experiences. The idea is to help the children to process what they are doing. There is also spontaneous reflection on the part of the children in groups. The cottage chat is a similar type of reflection and these are guided reflections during the evenings. None of the other camps facilitate this time in the evening in their schedule for the group to come together and talk about what's happened.

It is interesting that none of the American camps utilise the precise order of Therapeutic Recreation. The invariant order of Therapeutic Recreation is not explicit in the Painted Turtle though the camp activities are similar. In the Painted Turtle they follow a behaviour model called the STAR: Stay safe, Try something new, Always build up, Respect everybody. The campers sign up to the STAR model at the beginning of the camp. Both campers and counselors are aware of the STAR code, whereas the mantras of Therapeutic Recreation are known only to the Caras and the support staff at Barretstown and the European camps. These apparent differences between Barretstown and the Painted Turtle are superficial in terms of the camping experience. The Therapeutic Recreation framework is helpful to volunteers in Europe, as there is less tradition of the camping lifestyle, but the grammar of a four-step mnemonic is unnecessary for old camping hands in the USA. Therapeutic recreation is a useful short hand for the ethos of camping, which is unfamiliar to most Europeans. In practice, the European camps are more muted than their American counterparts, but they both have a common temporal and spatial structure with an emphasis on communitas and social efficacy that is impervious to the instrumental concerns of the world.

Serious Fun camps in Europe

Serious Fun camps have a detailed method of assessing facilities and practices in camps that are members of the association. Camps are inspected every two years based on their camping programmes and medical facilities. The process consists of detailed questionnaires supplemented by examination of their amenities. Both the French and the UK camps had sub-optimal reports from previous visits. The shortcomings of the UK and the French camps can now be analysed, understood and corrected with the paradigm that therapeutic benefits of Serious Fun camps are derived from their being structured in the form of a rite of passage. The sub-optimal outcomes found in the 2009 reports of the UK and the French camps were essentially structural problems in the sense that their anthropological rite of passage structure was compromised.

The evidence from Serious Fun camps suggests that an optimal therapeutic outcome depends on a structured experience of a rite of passage, consisting of three distinct stages: a stage of separation, a liminal stage characterised by communitas and a stage of re-integration. The sub-optimal experience of the French and the English camps could be redressed if there was better appreciation of the importance of a rite of passage structure. The French camp L'Envol (taking flight) was subsidised by their government, but in return the camp was required to serve many medical conditions. The camp was effectively a tertiary care children's hospital linked to a camping facility. The medical complexity of several difficult conditions demanded close medical supervision of the children at the camp. The children stayed in small dormitories in the chateau. There was a medical facility like a nurse's station adjacent to the bedrooms. The L'Envol experience, unlike the Barretstown experience, was not a sequestered rite of passage as there was no separation from hospital facilities. Links with home could be maintained by an easily available public telephone, unlike Barretstown, where there are no phone or social media links with the outside world. The requirement that L'Envol should provide a service for many medical conditions of tertiary paediatric care introduced a medical complexity that was ever present. The medical presence there could not be confined to a 'med shed'. This was an insoluble problem as long as L'Envol was required to take many complex medical conditions at the same time. Our suggested solution as visiting assessors was to adopt a service like the Painted Turtle, which caters for a single medical condition on a weekly basis – that worked for the most difficult medical conditions except for diabetes mellitus as at intervals the counselors had to adopt medical responsibilities.

The structural problems for the UK camp (Over the Wall) were slightly different although also a failure to achieve the necessary strong degree of separation for a clearly structured rite of passage as Over the Wall had to share their facility with other voluntary organisations. As a result, there was easy access to the outside world. Over the Wall does not have its own grounds, so that it must hire and share property with other associations. Separation and communitas are incomplete. Many of the cohabiting societies are like-minded, but the sharing does intrude and this can be seen in the relatively tame interaction in the communal dining halls. The problem is two-fold: First, there is no effective separation from the outside world as the property is not 'exclusive' in the positive sociological–anthropological sense. It is not an exclusive symbolic space identified as a 'sacred' zone set apart for ritual transformations and separate from profane routines in the everyday of home and hospital. The other camps have an exclusive identity as Barretstown is a castle, the Painted Turtle is an African village and L'Envol is a chateau – even if the latter fails to exclude the hospital dimension. Castles and chateaux are simulacra of African villages: they are 'magical' or 'sacred' spaces – spaces that are very different and distinct from the multi-use facility, where Over the Wall is situated. The second difficulty with the UK camp is the existence of several diverse groups of people within the same space, for example, healthy campers and sick children, whose different usages of the facilities are taking place simultaneously: Boy Scouts and other youth groups confuse the common experience of seriously ill children who are a very particular cohort. Sick children have a shared experience of hospitals and serious illness that triggers the safety of mutual recognition which is essential to their experience of communitas. The Barretstown experience suggests that both French and British camps could be improved by structural alterations: the French camp needs to simplify the medical aspect, which can be done by limiting each camp session to a single medical condition; the UK camp would benefit from not sharing the amenity with healthy campers.

Tripartite experiences

All the camps have a rite of passage structure to a greater or lesser degree. The degree that camps conform to the classical rite of passage structure may impact the beneficial effects of camps. The discovered principles of classical rites of passage should be adhered to as far as possible to optimise social changes. These are as follows:

1   Stage I: separation – separation from the real world must be strong, clear and unambiguous: a significant passage from the profane to the sacred.

2   Stage II: liminality – there must be intense communitas that encourages openness to change in liminal situations. The stage must entail a significant challenge suited to the child's condition and abilities. It must culminate in a meaningful achievement recognised and applauded by fellow campers. The stage of liminality must be supervised by wise and experienced Masters of Ceremonies who ensure success.

3   Stage III: re-integration – there must be deliberate and careful preparation for return to home and hospital. This can be achieved in rest times by structured conversations and reflections in their cabins or cottages led by their Caras or Counselors. Before going home the campers need to imagine their transformed selves in different settings, when they re-enter the real world.

The degree of separation in L'Envol and Over the Wall was quite incomplete. Over the Wall was hardly separate because of its proximity to other societies and the outside world. The contact with other organisations and the ease of exit made a rite of separation very difficult to sustain. L'Envol had a telephone beside the dining hall that allowed campers to phone home. All modern electronic paraphernalia including mobile phones are forbidden in Barretstown and the Painted Turtle. The ease of phoning home in the French camp is in striking contrast to the Painted Turtle, where there is a designated person, the Turtle Whisperer, to trouble shoot home sickness. Missing home tends to only occur in the first couple of days of the camp and there is a sophisticated graded response to children who are upset. Children who overcome home sickness tend to have a brilliant experience and are often amongst the most tearful when the camp has ended. There have been rare situations when children have had to be flown home early because of missing home. The medical presence is formidable in L'Envol compared with the almost dumbing down of the medical input in Barretstown (the med shed – the terminology is perfect). The Well Shell in the Painted Turtle is a superb facility brilliantly disguised as part of the African village style set up of camp. The proximity of medical facilities to bedrooms in L'Envol makes separation from the hospital world impossible. The lack of separation from the real world is also evident in the retention of titles such as professor and doctor, which was apparent in both L'Envol and Over the Wall, whereas everyone is addressed by their first names only at the Hole in the Wall, the Painted Turtle and Barretstown.

The intensity of social interaction is important for change and facilitated by what Victor Turner calls communitas. This is an atmosphere of I–thou relationships in the interaction amongst the children and with their Cara/Counselors that becomes special and life transforming. It is very evident in Barretstown and the Painted Turtle and facilitated there by dancing and singing at mealtimes. The indicators of communitas at Barretstown are participation in dancing and singing in the dining hall. There is a gradual take-up of dancing from day one as the children lose their inhibitions of the outside world. This seems to take about three days. Different and important social interactions take place in the cottages or cabins. I learn of this only by hear-say because they are private and personal between Caras and children, but cottage chats are undoubtedly important as a confidential site of close com-munication. What is said in the cottages stays in the cottages. In both L'Envol and Over the Wall, the level of social interaction at mealtimes seemed muted compared to the camps with a complete rite of passage structure. Despite these drawbacks the achievements of both camps are formidable.

Serious Fun International: creative adaptation

Serious Fun camps have responded to pressing concerns in different countries. Sibling neglect is often an unintended consequence in families looking after a child with cancer. Sibling camps were one of the first innovations. These camps are very demanding as the children are healthy but anxious about their health. Medical facilities are busier during a sibling session than camps for their sick brothers and sisters. Kinsella et al. (2006) made the interesting observation that siblings made greater use of the medical facility than their brothers or sisters with cancer. Hanlon et al. (2016) have been instrumental in setting up the Barretstown Bereavement programme for families whose child died from a serious illness. This programme has been much appreciated by parents and their families. Professionals from the Hole in the Wall Gang Camp have sought to replicate this programme in Connecticut reversing the transatlantic direction of expertise. Serious Fun International has spread be-yond Europe to Israel and Japan. In a different way, the Global Partnership Program offers camp experiences to children living with serious illnesses in Africa, Asia and the Caribbean by cooperating with local programmes.

Conclusion

The experiences of Serious Fun campers and their carers suggest that challenging events in a Rite of Passage structure are salutogenic when monitored by exemplary Masters of Ceremonies. Serious Fun camps are modern institutions that have a social structure in common with ancient rites of passage. The benefits of these ancient and modern practices must be more than a coincidence. Salutogenic social transformations are best achieved when guided by Masters of Ceremonies in a ritual process of separation, transitional liminality and reintegration anew back to society.

> 'When I use a *word*,' Humpty Dumpty said, in rather a scornful tone, 'it *means* just what I *choose* it to *mean* – neither more nor less.'
>
> Lewis Carroll: *Alice in Wonderland*

In an era of fake news, Humpty Dumpty seems to have regained control of the lexicon. Words appear inefficient and even misleading. The quiet desperation of social suffering persists despite proffered remedies of mindfulness, resilience and equality. In 2017, the seventh international conference on the Social Pathologies of Contemporary Civilization was held in Frankfort to explore the nature of social suffering in an era of resilience. The diseases to be explored were stress-related disorders of the collective *esprit de corps* such as anxiety, depression and substance abuse. Solutions to problems of the collective may need institutional reforms in the domains of politics, law, religion and economics and not a focus on improving an individual's resilience. Resilience is very much in vogue as an attribute that can resist the social pathologies of our contemporary world. Resilience may help a bit, but, in effect, it distracts humanity from exploring more relevant and ambitious solutions at social and cultural levels. This book hints that salutogenesis may be a more appropriate antidote to the current malaise of social pathology. In a way resilience can be part of salutogenesis as a natural resource (an innate ability to bend but not break) that Antonovsky could have included under general resistance resources (GRR). These GRR, together with social experiences that improve an individual's sense of coherence, contrive to promote salutogenesis.

Salutogenesis is a social process captured by the metaphor of learning to swim in the river of life. It is no use building bridges (avoiding all stress) so that we do not fall into the river (Eriksson, 2007). River swimming implies engagement with risk and life's uncertainties. We are heterostatic creatures. We seek new experiences that may transform our being for better or worse. Salutogenesis is about the generation of health and includes both physical and social health, but it is primarily social as 'the pursuit of health and happiness is guided by urges that are social rather than biological' (Dubos, 1995). The experiences of Serious Fun campers and their carers suggest that challenging experiences in a rite of passage structure are salutogenic when monitored by exemplary Masters of Ceremonies (MCs) as adepts. Children with cancer and leukaemia are unavoidably separated from their peers and families by treatment of the illness and its harmful consequences. They were the first group of children to benefit from the Serious Fun experience. Serious Fun camps now cater for many serious childhood illnesses including disabilities. The benefit accruing to these children does not directly impact their physical illnesses. The benefit is social, which may translate into better outcomes through improved compliance with treatments. Could these benefits transform children with the classical problems of social pathology such as anxiety, depression and related mental disorders? It remains to be seen, but the effect on children with serious childhood illnesses is a psycho–social transformation towards healthful engagement with the world. The Beslan High School siege in 2004 resulted in the massacre of over 350 children and adults. The crisis played out over three days in September and horrified the world. Countries and charities donated funds to assist families and children involved in the crisis including an Irish charity (Deegan, 2012). As a result, some of the survivors were funded for a holiday in Barretstown. It is not known whether their intervention made a difference to the survivors – many of whom would have had post-traumatic stress disorder, but six years later there is a clue in a line from an email to the organiser of the holiday in Barretstown. A mother of a Beslan siege survivor writes:

> We remember every minute of our stay in Ireland. It was you who returned our children back to life.
>
> (Deegan, 2012)

The idea of deliberate interventions for the ills of social pathology is sound and merits further exploration.

According to Girard et al. (2007), we stumble on social processes such as the sacrificial mechanism by accident, and that also seems to have been the case with healing rites of passage in Serious Fun camps. Girard suggested that the burgeoning intelligence of evolving humanity fuelled by increasing imitative skills was put at risk by violent rivalry. That is until hominids were jolted into self-awareness by the shock of an innocent victim – the scapegoat's cadaver. The mechanism delivered peace and so the scapegoat became a saviour. That social process according to Girard was the foundation of all religions, cultures and institutions. The discovery of effective social processes can be sustained by ritual, myth and taboos. Ritual repeats and thereby recalls the process, which is then mythologised in legends that cloud ancestral guilt of the scapegoat murder, while taboos are placed on the triggering circumstances of mutual assured destruction. It is a story, but a good suggestion of how we became self-aware. It is also the story of the foundation of Serious Fun camps as the founders stumbled by accident on the social process of salutogenesis in healing rites of passage. The American camp experience was in place for over a century when the Hole in the Wall Gang Camp opened in 1988. Simple modifications to that experience introduced new possibilities for seriously ill children. Newman's vision was of a place where the illness could be effectively sidelined for a while: 'I just wanted a place where children could raise a little hell', but it proved to be much more than a respite from intensive hospital treatments. Beneficial social transformations were an accidental outcome. Newman and his team had stumbled on a process of salutogenesis in conditions resembling tribal rites of passage. The word spread in the small world of Paediatric Oncology in America and then across the Atlantic. According to Gerard, our forefathers stumbled on the social process of the scapegoat mechanism, which rescued our species from self-destruction; but the founding myth that veiled ancestral guilt was slowly revealed in the Bible as murder of an innocent victim. As Nietzsche said, 'God is dead, and we have killed him'. Sacred rituals of the saviour no longer convince, and taboos no longer restrain mimetic violence. Murder of the innocents as in Beslan still appals, but the media has sanitised and insulated the reality of killing and dying. Salutogenic rites of passage are a social process for the twenty-first century. They will not establish new religions but they can generate healthful world views. They are a small-scale solution to stress-related disorders.

Rites of passage govern social change by acknowledging elevation of social status or resisting change by the ridicule of social reversal (Turner, 1969). After camp the children's medical health was in status quo. They were still sick children. The transformation was in their social being. There is trouble with words in trying to understand the distinction of genesis and mimesis. Genesis, genes and genetics link to the unfolding of Darwin's evolutionary change. Mimesis links to the power of social interaction in cultural transmission and Lamarck's inheritance of acquired characteristics. There is no hint of mimesis in the etymology of sociogenesis, psychogenesis and salutogenesis, but in the adaptation to change the mimetic apparatus is at least as powerful as the genome in humanity. Darwin triumphed in the twentieth century, but the twenty first may belong to Lamarck through Girard's triangles of desire.

Paul Newman was well liked by men and women, but he was not a saint. He had a difficult relationship with his father, who died before he became an international film star. Newman in turn had an offhand relationship with his own son Scott, who found it difficult to deal with his father's fame.

The author A.E. Hotchner and Paul Newman had a great friendship, which Hotchner (2011) describes in an affectionate memoir. Hotchner does not shy away from Newman's troubled relationship with his son from his first marriage. Newman was an absentee father while his teenage son ran into all sorts of social difficulties. Newman admitted to Hotchner that there was a failure of communication between father and son. Newman had 'lined up a shrink' for Scott, who did not seem to have any friends and resorted to various substance abuses. Paul Newman confided in Hotchner after Scott died aged twenty-eight from an overdose of drugs and alcohol:

> Scott died before he had a fair chance to be a success...at something. I think about him...often...it hurts. The guilt. The guilt. All I could have done... and didn't do.
>
> (Hotchner, 2011:78)

It was a tragedy that could not be reversed. Paul Newman was not an exemplary prophet, but he was able to learn from his mistakes. His absence from the trials and tribulation of his son did not prevent him from being an ethical prophet with an inchoate vision of how to help seriously ill children.

Salutogenesis is a word that is slowly gaining traction as an important concept in the social sciences. It is unlikely that Paul Newman had ever heard of the word before he died in 2008, but he was certainly aware of good luck. Antonovsky's neologism of salutogenesis crystallises Newman's vague sense of what he wanted to achieve for seriously ill children. He understood his personal health, wealth and happiness as a matter of luck and how his gifts bestowed by chance could help generate good times by sharing spoils with the less fortunate (Hotchner, 2011). The genesis of *salut* is towards a holistic form of health. It includes the universal toast of good luck amongst well-wishers in thanksgiving for the gift of friendship, health and well-being. 'Good Luck' acknowledges uncertainty into the future whilst accepting gratitude for the present. Paul Newman always attributed his inspiration for the Hole in the Wall Gang Camp as a matter of luck. He instinctively understood the gift economy propelled by charity and its distinction from the market. Newman made a lot of money from films, but his venture into the food business was even more successful. It started almost as a lark with a friend but evolved into a very successful commercial operation. His philosophy was summarised by the company motto of 'shameless exploitation in pursuit of the common good'. All profits from Newman's Own are donated to charity and along with a generous gift from the Royal Kingdom of Saudi Arabia helped establish the Hole in the Wall Gang Camp (Pearson and Shefsky, 2016). Paul Newman's biography shows a long-term commitment to political ideals. He was guided by a deep awareness of injustice informed by his own good luck of being blessed with talent, good looks and an engaging personality. His awareness of bad luck in others was perhaps sensitised by his dysfunctional relationship with his son and epitomised by the misfortunes of seriously ill children. When asked what he would like to be remembered for, he ignored his cinematic achievements and always answered 'the camps'.

The inspiration for this book came from children attending a leukaemia clinic, who had been subdued by treatment and then appeared transformed by a short holiday in Barretstown. Social transformations are not in the lexicon of Paediatric practice. Volunteering there as a Paediatrician with a late vocation to Sociology convinced me that the transforming powers of Barretstown are compatible with healing rites of passage. Barretstown is a sophisticated operation and it took a visit to the USA to understand how Serious Fun camps came into being. They are the product of fine tuning the American summer camp experience. The assembly of that experience has emerged with attributes of ancient rites of passage. The benefits of these ancient and modern practices suggest their common structure must be more than a coincidence. These ritual processes are universal to all cultures. Social transformations guided by MCs are best achieved by separation, transitional liminality and re-integration anew. MCs (Caras and Counselors) hold the key as they model an ideal of well-being, which can be subconsciously imitated in the magical liminality of Serious Fun camps. Rites of passage traditionally celebrate transformation of social status. Serious Fun camps have, without realising it, adapted that ritual experience as the ideal circumstance for trans-forming the social health of children accidentally stigmatised by chronic life-threatening illnesses. The black and white magic of ritual was demeaned by eighteenth-century Enlightenment philosophers. Medical science had to replace the healing rituals of witchcraft. The importance of liminal experi-ences for social change and recovery were reinstated by Arnold van Gennep and Victor Turner in the twentieth century through their recognition of rites of passage. The lawless nature of liminality with its sense of the uncanny, trepidation, excitement and opportunity can produce the white magic of benign social transformations when marshalled by exemplary MCs – the Caras and the Counselors of Serious Fun camps. The transformation process is not without risk as Tricksters posing as MCs can corrupt social change towards the black magic of envy, rivalry and violence. The white magic of salutogenesis orientates personal beliefs towards a sense of personal, social and cultural coherence. The world can be understood, revealing existence as meaningful because there are resources available to navigate the predictable and unpredictable passage ways in our journey through life.

References

Albrecht, G. L. and P. J. Devlieger (1999). "The Disability Paradox: High Quality of Life Against All Odds." *Social Science & Medicine* **48**(8): 977–988.

Alexander, J. (1987). *Twenty Lectures: Sociological Theory Since World War II*. New York, Columbia University Press.

Antonovsky, A. (1979). *Health, Stress and Coping*. San Franciso, CA, Jossey-Bass Publishers.

Antonovsky, A. (1987). *Unravelling the Mystery of Health: How People Manage Stress and Stay Well*. San Francisco, CA, Jossey-Bass Publishers.

Antonovsky, A. (1990). "A Somewhat Personal Odyssey in Studying the Stress Process." *Stress Medicine* **6**: 71–80.

Antonovsky, A. and S. Sagy (2017). "Aaron Antonovsky, the Scholar and the Man Behind Salutogenesis." *The Handbook of Salutogenesis*. M. B. Mittelmark, M. Eriksson, J. M. Pelikan et al. Springer: 461.

Arnett, J. J. (2006). G. Stanley Hall's Adolescence: Brilliance and nonsense. *History of Psychology* **9**(3), 186–197.

Aronson, J. K. (2006). "Autopathography: The Patient's Tale." *British Medical Journal* **321**: 1599–1602.

Astell, A. W. (2004). "Saintly Mimesis, Contagion, and Empathy in the Thought of René Girard, Edith Stein, and Simone Weil." *Shofar: An Interdisciplinary Journal of Jewish Studies* **22**(2): 116–131.

Baden-Powell, R. (2007). *Playing the Game. A Baden-Powell Compendium*. Oxford, Macmillan.

Baer, L. and W. Gesler (2004). "Reconsidering the Concept of Therapeutic Landscapes in JD Salinger's *The Catcher in the Rye*." *Area* **36**(4): 404–413.

Bauby, J. -D. (2008). *The Diving-Bell and the Butterfly*. London, HarperCollins Publishers.

Beecher, S. (1991). *A Dictionary of Cork Slang*. Cork, The Collins Press.

Bekesi, A., S. Torok et al. (2011). "Health-related Quality of Life Changes of Children and Adolescents with Chronic Disease After Participation in Therapeutic Recreation Camping Program." *Health and Quality of Life Outcomes* **9**(42): 1–10.

Berntson, G. G. and J. T. Cacioppo (2007). "Integrative Physiology: Homeostasis, Allostasis and the Orchestration of Systemic Physiology." *Handbook of Psychophysiology*. G. Tassinary and G. Berntson. Cambridge, Cambridge University Press: 433–452.

Bhakta, N., K. K. Ness et al. (2017). "The Cumulative Burden of Surviving Childhood Cancer: An Initial Report from the St Jude Lifetime Cohort Study (SJLIFE)." *Lancet* **390**(10112): 2569–2582.

128   *References*

Black, D., J. N. Morris et al. (1988). *Inequalities in Health, the Black Report and the Health Divide*. London, Pelican Books.

Bruno, M.-A., J. L. Bernheim et al. (2011). "A Survey on Self-assessed Well-being in a Cohort of Chronic Locked-in Syndrome Patients: Happy Majority, Miserable Minority." *BMJ Open* **1**(1): e000039.

Canguilhem, G. (1991). *The Normal and the Pathological*. New York, Zone Books.

Carlson, K. P. and M. Cook (2007). "Challenge by Choice: Adventure-Based Counseling for Seriously Ill Adolescents." *Child and Adolescent Psychiatric Clinics of North America* **16**: 909–919.

Clark, A. (1997). *Being There: Putting Brain, Body, and World Together Again*. Cambridge, MA, The MIT Press.

Collins, N. (2001). "Don Imus on His Mexico Ranch." *Architectural Digest. The International Magazine of Interior Design*.

Csikszentmihalyi, M. (1991). *Flow: The Psychology of Optimal Experience*. New York, Harper Perennial.

Dearn, A. (2006). *The Hitler Youth 1933–45*. Osprey Publishing.

Deegan, D. (2012). "Joe Duffy, Barretstown and Beslan." *To Russia with Love*. Cork, Mercier Press.

Deflem, M. (1991). "Ritual, Antistructure, and Religion: A Discussion of Victor Turner's Processual Symbolic Analysis." *Journal for the Scientific Study of Religion* **30**(1): 1–25.

Doble, J., A. Haig et al. (2003). "Impairment, Activity, Participation, Life Satisfaction and Survival in Persons with Locked-in Syndrome for Over a Decade." *J Head Trauma Rehabil* **5**: 434–444.

Dolan, P. and B. Brady (2011). *A Guide to Youth Mentoring. Providing Effective Social Support*. London, Jessica Kingsley.

Donald, M. (1991). *Origins of the Modern Mind. Three Stages in the Evolution of Culture and Cognition*. Cambridge, MA, Harvard University Press.

Donald, M. (2005). "Imitation and Mimesis." *Perspectives on Imitation – From Neuroscience to Social Science*. S. Hurley and N. Chater. London, The MIT Press. 2: Imitation, Human Development and Culture: 283–300.

Dubos, R. (1959/1988). *Mirage of Health*. New Brunswick, NJ, Rutgers University Press.

Durkheim, E. (1995). *The Elementary Forms of Religious Life*. New York, The Free Press.

Eiser, C. (2004). *Children with Cancer: The Quality of Life*. Mahwah, NJ, Lawrence Erlbaum Associates.

Eiser, C. and M. Jenney (2007). "Measuring Quality of Life." *Arch Dis Child* **92**: 348–350.

Elias, N. (2000). *The Civilizing Process*. Oxford, Blackwell Publishing.

Eriksson, M. (2007). *Unravelling the Mystery of Salutogenesis*. Helsinki, Folkhalsan Research Centre.

Eriksson, M. and B. Lindström (2011). "Life is More Than Survival: Exploring Links Between Antonovsky's Salutogenic Theory and the Concept of Resilience." *Way Finding Through Life's Challenges: Coping and Survival*. K. Gow and M. J. Celinski. New York, Nova Science Publishers Inc.: 31–46.

Gately, P. J., C. B. Cooke et al. (2005). "Children's Residential Weight-Loss Programs Can Work: A Prospective Cohort Study for Overweight and Obese Children." *Pediatrics* **116**(1): 73–77.

Farber, S., L. K. Diamond et al. (1948). "Temporary Remissions in Acute Leukemia in Children Produced by Folic Acid Antagonist, 4-Aminopteroly-glutamic acid (Aminopterin)." *N Eng J Med* **238**(23): 787–793.

Frei III, E., E. J. Freireich et al. (1961). "Studies of Sequential and Combination Antimetabolite Therapy in Acute Leukemia: 6-Mercaptopurine and Methotrexate." *Blood* **18**: 431–454.

Gadamer, H. -G. (1996). *The Enigma of Health*. Stanford, CA, Stanford University Press.

Gaffney, A., B. Morris et al. (2006). "Family Benefits of a Local Service in Paediatric Oncology." *Arch Dis Child* **91**(Suppl 1): 82.

Gallese, V. (2009). "The Two Sides of Mimesis. Girard's Mimetic Theory, Embodied Simulation and Social Identification." *Journal of Consciousness Studies* **16**(4): 1–24.

Gesler, W. and R. Kearns (2002). "Landscapes of Healing." *Culture/Place/Health*. London, Routledge: 120–138.

Girard, R. (1977). *Violence and the Sacred*. Baltimore, MD, The Johns Hopkins University Press.

Girard, R. (1996). "Triangular Desire." *The Girard Reader*. J. G. Williams. New York, The Crossroad Publishing Company: 33–44.

Girard, R., P. Antonello et al. (2007). *Evolution and Conversion*. London, Bloomsbury Academic.

Goffman, E. (1990). *Stigma. Notes on the Management of Spoiled Identity*. London, Penguin Books Ltd.

Goffman, E. (1997). "The Mortified Self." *The Goffman Reader*. C. Lemert and A. Branaman. Oxford, Blackwell Publishing: 55–71.

Green, G. (2009). *The End of Stigma. Changes in the Social Experience of Long-Term Illness*. London, Routledge.

Gurney, J. G., K. R. Krull et al. (2009). "Social Outcomes in the Childhood Cancer Survivor Study Cohort." *Journal of Clinical Oncology* **27**(14): 2390–2395.

Hall, G. S. (1904). *Adolescence: Its Psychology and Its Relations to Physiology, Anthropology, Sociology, Sex, Crime, Religion, and Education*. New York, D. Appleton and Co.

Hamerton-Kelly, R. (1992). Eros and Agape. *Sacred Violence: Paul's Hermeneutic of the Cross*. Minneapolis, MN, Augsburg Fortress: 161–173.

Handelman, D. (1998). *Models and Mirrors Towards an Anthropology of Public Events*. New York, Berghahn Books.

Hanlon, P., S. Guerin et al. (2016). "Supporting Parents Who Have Lost a Child to Serious Illness: Combining Bereavement and Therapeutic Recreation Models of Intervention." *Pediatric Blood and Cancer* **63**: S226–S226.

Hardisty, R. M., M. M. Till et al. (1981). "Acute Lymphoblastic Leukaemia: Four-Year Survivals Old and New." *Journal of Clinical Pathology* **34**: 249–253.

Heath, J. A., N. E. Clarke et al. (2010). "Symptoms and Suffering at the End of Life in Children with Cancer: An Australian Perspective." *MJA* **192**(2): 71–75.

Hewitt, M., S. L. Weiner et al. (2003). "The Epidemiology of Childhood Cancer." *Childhood Cancer Survivorship Improving Care and Quality of Life*. M. Hewitt, S. L. Weiner and J. V. Simone. Washington, DC, The National Academies Press: 20–36.

Holloman, R. E. (1974). "Ritual Opening and Individual Transformation: Rites of Passage at Esalen." *American Anthropologist* **76**(2): 265–280.

Holmes, T. H. and R. H. Rahe (1967). "The Social Readjustment Rating Scale." *Journal of Psychosomatic Research* **11**(2): 213–218.

Hoopes, J. (1991). *Peirce on Signs. Writings on Semiotics by Charles Sanders Peirce*. Chapel Hill, University of North Carolina.

Horvath, A. and B. Thomassen (2008). "Mimetic Errors in Liminal Schismogenesis: On the Political Anthropology of the Trickster." *International Political Anthropology* **1**(1): 3–24.

Hotchner, A. E. (2011). *Paul and Me. 53 Years of Adventures and Misadventures with My Pal Paul Newman.* New York, Anchor Books.

Huizinga, J. (1955). *Homo Ludens: A Study of the Play Elements in Culture.* Boston, MA, Beacon Press.

Hurley, S. and N. Chater (2005). *Perspectives on Imitation: From Neuroscience to Social Science.* Cambridge, MA, The MIT Press.

Hyde, L. (2007). *The Gift. Creativity and the Artist in the Modern World.* New York, Vintage Books.

Kearney, P. J. (1976). "Personal View." *British Medical Journal* **1**: 1069.

Kearney, P. J. (2006). "Autopathography and Humane Medicine: The Diving Bell and the Butterfly – An Interpretation." *Medical Humanities* **32**: 111–113.

Kearney, P. J. (2009). "The Barretstown Experience: A Rite of Passage." *Irish Journal of Sociology* **17**(2): 72–89.

Kearns, R. and D. Collins (2000). "New Zealand Children's Health Camps: Therapeutic Landscape Meets the Contract State." *Social Science and Medicine* **50**: 1047–1059.

Keel, B. (2005). "The Imus Ranch Helping Children." *American Profile.*

Kempe, C. H., F. N. Silverman et al. (1962). "The Battered-Child Syndrome." *JAMA* **181**(1): 17–24.

Keohane, K. and C. Kuhling (2014). "Conversion: Turning Towards a Radiant Ideal." *The Domestic Moral and Political Economies of Post-Celtic Tiger Ireland. What Rough Beast?* Manchester, Manchester University Press: 107–122.

Keohane, K., A. Petersen et al. (2017). "Introduction to a Series." *Late Modern Subjectivity and Its Discontents.* K. Keohane, A. Petersen and B. van den Bergh. London, Routledge.

Kiernan, G., M. Gormley et al. (2004). "Outcomes Associated with Participation in a Therapeutic Recreation Camping Programme for Children from 15 European Countries: Data from the 'Barretstown Studies'." *Social Science & Medicine* **59**: 903–913.

Kiernan, G. and M. MacLachlan (2002). "Children's Perspectives of Therapeutic Recreation: Data from the 'Barretstown Studies'." *J of Health Psychology* **7**(5): 599–613.

Kinsella, E., P. Zeltzer et al. (2006). "Safety of Summer Camp for Children with Chronic and/or Life Threatening Illness." *European Journal of Oncology Nursing* **10**(4): 304–310.

Klopf, A. (1972). *Brain Function and Adaptive Systems: A Heterostatic Theory.* Bedford, MA, Air Force Cambridge Research Laboratories.

Korotkov, D. (1998). "The Sense of Coherence: Making Sense Out of Chaos." *A Handbook of Psychological Research and Clinical Applications.* P. T. Wong and P. S. Fry. Mahwah, NJ, Lawrence Erlbaum Associates: 51–70.

Krueger, G. M. (2007). "For Jimmy and the Boys and Girls of America": Publicizing Childhood Cancers in Twentieth Century America." *Bulletin of the History of Medicine* **8**(1): 70–93.

Kuhn, T. S. (1996). *The Structure of Scientific Revolutions.* Chicago, IL, The University of Chicago Press.

Langeveld, N. E., M. A. Grootenhuis et al. (2004). "Posttraumatic Stress Symptoms in Adult Survivors of Childhood Cancer." *Pediatr Blood Cancer* **42**(7): 604–610.

Larcombe, I., M. Mott et al. (2002). "Lifestyle Behaviours of Young Adult Survivors of Childhood Cancer." *British Journal of Cancer* **87**: 1204–1209.

Larcombe, I., J. Walker et al. (1990). "Impact of Childhood Cancer on Return to Normal Schooling." *BMJ* **301**: 169–171.

Last, J. M. (1997). *Public Health and Human Ecology.* McGraw-Hill Medical.

Lerner, B. H. (2010). "A Doctor Goes to Cancer Camp." New York, *The New York Times.*

Lutz, J. (2009). "Flow and Sense of Coherence: Two Aspects of the Same Dynamic?" *Global Health Promotion* **16**(3): 63–67.

Malafouris, L. (2013). *How Things Shape the Mind. A Theory of Material Engagement.* Cambridge, MA, The MIT Press.

Mandela, N. (1994). *The Long Walk to Freedom. The Autobiography of Nelson Mandela.* London, Little Brown and Company.

Masten, A. S. and A. H. Gewirtz (2006). "Vulnerability and Resilience in Early Child Development." *Blackwell Handbook of Early Childhood Development.* K. McCartney and D. Phillips. Oxford, Blackwell Publishing Ltd: 663.

McAuliffe-Fogarty, A. H., R. Ramsing et al. (2007). "Medical Specialty Camps for Youth with Diabetes." *Child and Adolescent Psychiatric Clinics of North America.* A. H. McAuliffe-Fogarty and K. P. Carlson. Philadelphia, PA, Saunders. **16**: 887–908.

McNamara, J. (2009). "American Genesis: Nationalism's Secular Hierophany." *Sociology.* Cork, University College Cork: 272.

Meltzoff, A. N. and M. K. Moore (1977). "Imitation of Facial and Manual Gestures by Human Neonates." *Science* **198**(4312): 75–8.

Mercer, R. D. (1999). "The Team." *Medical and Pediatric Oncology* **33**: 407–408.

Merrill, T. C. (2013). *The Book of Imitation and Desire. Reading Milan Kundera with René Girard.* London, Bloomsbury Publishing Plc.

Meyler, E., S. Guerin et al. (2010). "Review of Family-Based Psychosocial Interventions for Childhood Cancer." *Journal of Pediatric Psychology* **35**(10): 1116–1132.

Mittelmark, M. B., S. Sagy et al. (2017). *The Handbook of Salutogenesis.* Springer.

Mukherjee, S. (2010). *The Emperor of all Maladies. A Biography of Cancer.* New York, Scribner.

NICE (2005). *Post-Traumatic Stress Disorder: The Management of PTSD in Adults and Children in Primary and Secondary Care.* London, Gaskell and the British Psychological Society: 1–41.

Nussbaum, M. and A. Sen (1993). "Introduction." *The Quality of Life.* M. Nussbaum and A. Sen. Oxford, Oxford University Press: 1–6.

Oeffinger, K. C., A. C. Mertens et al. (2006). "Chronic Health Conditions in Adult Survivors of Childhood Cancer." *N Eng J Med* **355**: 1572–1582.

Oughourlian, J. M. (2016). *The Mimetic Brain.* East Lansing, Michigan State University Press.

Palaver, W. (2013). *Rene Girard's Mimetic Theory.* East Lansing, Michigan State University Press.

Parsons, T. (1951). *The Social System.* London, Routledge & Kegan Paul Ltd.

Patenaude, A. F. and M. J. Kupst (2005). "Psychosocial Functioning in Pediatric Cancer." *Journal of Pediatric Psychology* **30**(1): 9–27.

Pearson, H. A. and M. L. Shefsky (2015). *Doc's Story. The Hole in the Wall Gang Camp and Its Totem Poles.* New Haven, CT, www.holeinthewallgang.org.

Pearson, H. A. and M. L. Shefsky (2016). *Fulfilling Paul Newman's Dream.* Seattle, WA, Lookbook Press.

Pelikan, J. M. (2017). "The Application of Salutogenesis in Healthcare Settings." *The Handbook of Salutogenesis.* M. B. Mittelmark, S. Sagy, M. Eriksson et al. Springer Nature: 261–263.

Peterson, C. A. and N. J. Stumbo (2000). *Therapeutic Recreation Programme Design: Principles and Procedures.* Boston, MA, Allyn and Bacon.

Rappaport, R. A. (1999). *Ritual and Religion in the Making of Humanity.* Cambridge, Cambridge University Press.

Rivera, G., D. Pinkel et al. (1993). "Treatment of Acute Lymphoblastic Leukemia. 30 Years' Experience at St Jude Children's Research Hospital." *N Engl J Med* **329**: 1289–1295.

Scheper-Hughes, N. (2014). "The House Gun. White Writing, White Fears and Black Justice." *Anthropology Today* **30**(6): 8–12

Schou, K. C. and J. Hewison (1999). *Experiencing Cancer: Quality of Life in Treatment (Facing Death).* Buckingham, Open University Press.

Selye, H. (1973). "Homeostasis and Heterostasis." *Perspectives in Biology and Medicine* **16**: 441–445.

Smith, M. A., N. L. Seibel et al. (2010). "Outcomes for Children and Adolescents with Cancer: Challenges for the Twenty-First Century." *Journal of Clinical Oncology* **28**(15): 2625–2634.

Smith, M. B. (2006). "'The Ego Ideal of the Good Camper' and the Nature of Summer Camp." *Environmental History* **11**(1): 70–101.

Sontag, S. (1991). *Illness as a Metaphor and Aids and Its Metaphors.* London, Penguin Books Ltd.

Spariosu, M. I. (1997). *The Wreath of Wild Olive. Play, Liminality, and the Study of Literature.* Albany, State University of New York Press.

Stam, H. (2005). "The Course of Life of Survivors of Childhood Cancer." *Psycho-Oncology* **14**: 227–238.

Szakolczai, A. (2000). *Reflexive Historical Sociolgy.* London, Routledge.

Szakolczai, A. (2003a). "Weber's Historical Method." *The Genesis of Modernity.* London, Routledge: 9–29.

Szakolczai, A. (2003b). "Ethical Prophecy." *The Genesis of Modernity.* London, Routledge: 30–48.

Szakolczai, A. (2010). "Masks and Persons: Identity Formation in Public." *International Political Anthropology* **3**(2): 171–191.

Szakolczai, A. (2013). "The Social Pathologies of Contemporary Civilization: Meaning-Giving Experiences and Pathological Expectations Concerning Health and Suffering." *The Social Pathologies of Contemporary Civilization.* K. Keohane and A. Petersen. Burlington, VT, Ashgate Publishing Company: 35–52.

Taieb, O., M. Moro et al. (2003). "Posttraumatic Stress Disorder After Childhood Cancer." *Eur Child Adolesc Psychiatry* **12**(6): 255–264.

Thomassen, B. (2014). *Liminality and the Modern. Living Through the In-Between.* Burlington, VT, Ashgate Publishing Limited.

Tominey, S. L., R. Pietrzak et al. (2015). "More Than Just Serious Fun: The Impact of Camp on Resilience for Campers with Serious Illness, Yale Child Study Centre."

Turner, V. (1969). *The Ritual Process: Structure and Antistructure.* New York, Aldine de Gruyter.

Turner, V. W. (1968). *The Drums of Affliction. Oxford, Oxford University Press.*

Turner, V. (1975). *Revelation and Divination in Ndembu Ritual.* Ithaca, NY, Cornell University Press.

Turner, V. (1980). "Social Dramas and Stories About Them." *Critical Inquiry* **7**(1): 141–168.

Turner, V. (1982). *From Ritual to Theatre the Human Seriousness of Play.* New York, PAJ Publications.

Turner, E. L. B. (1985). "Prologue: From the Ndembu to Broadway." *On the Edge of the Bush; Anthropology as Experience.* V. Turner and E. L. B. Turner. Tucson, The University of Arizona Press: 1–15.

Tusaie, K. and J. Dyer (2004). "Resilience: A Historical Review of the Construct." *Holistic Nursing Practice* **18**: 3–8.

van Gennep, A. (1960). *The Rites of Passage.* Chicago, IL, The University of Chicago Press.

Vinje, H. F., E. Langeland et al. (2017). "Aaron Antonovsky's Development of Salutogenesis, 1979 to 1994." *Handbook of Salutogenesis.* M. B. Mittelmark, S. Sagy, M. Eriksson et al. Springer: 25–40.

Vinje, H. F. and M. B. Mittelmark (2006). "Deflecting the Path to Burn-Out Among Community Health Nurses: How the Effective Practice of Self-Tuning Renews Job Engagement." *The International Journal of Mental Health Promotion* **8**(4): 36–47.

Walker, D. A. and D. Pearman (2009). "Therapeutic Recreation Camps: An Effective Intervention for Children and Young People with Chronic Illness?" *Arch Dis Child* **94**: 401–406.

Weber, M. (1978). "Basic Sociological Terms." *Economy and Society.* G. Roth and C. Wittich. Los Angeles, University of California Press: 3–62.

Whitehead, E., C. Carlisle et al. (2001). "Historical Developments." *Stigma and Social Exclusion in Healthcare.* T. Mason, C. Carlisle, C. Watkins and E. Whitehead. London, Routledge: 17–28.

WHO (1948). *Constitution of the World Health Organization.* Geneva, World Health Organization.

WHO (1984). "Health Promotion: A Discussion Document on the Concept and Principles: Summary Report of the Working Group on Concept and Principles of Health Promotion." Copenhagen, World Health Organization.

WHO (1986). "The Ottawa Charter for Health Promotion: An International Conference on Health Promotion, the Move Towards a New Public Health." Ottawa, World Health Organization.

Wikipedia (2017). Don Imus, Wikipedia. **2017**.

Wolfe, J., H. Grier et al. (2000). "Symptoms and Suffering at the End of Life in Children with Cancer." *N Eng J Med* **342**: 326–333.

Index

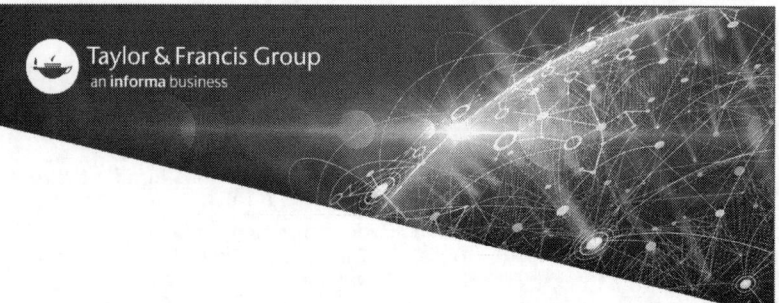
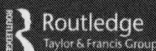
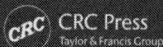